James Herriot's Favorite
DOG STORIES

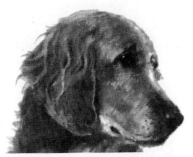

James Herriot's Favorite
DOG STORIES

James Herriot

With Illustrations by Lesley Holmes

G.K. Hall & Co. • **Chivers Press**
Thorndike, Maine USA   Bath, England

✓

This Large Print edition is published by G.K. Hall & Co., USA and by Chivers Press, England.

Published in 1997 in the U.S. by arrangement with St. Martin's Press, Inc.

Published in 1997 in the U.K. by arrangement with Michael Joseph Limited.

U.S. Hardcover	0-7838-1882-3	(Core Collection Edition)
U.K. Hardcover	0-7451-5410-7	(Windsor Large Print)
U.K. Softcover	0-7451-8722-6	(Paragon Large Print)

The text of this Large Print edition is unabridged.
Other aspects of the book may vary from the original edition.

Set in 18 pt. Bookman Old Style.

Printed in the United States on permanent paper.

British Library Cataloguing in Publication Data available

Library of Congress Cataloging in Publication Data
Herriot, James.
    [Favorite dog stories]
    James Herriot's favorite dog stories / with illustrations
by Lesley Holmes.
        p.   cm.
    ISBN 0-7838-1882-3 (lg. print : hc)
    1. Dogs — England — Yorkshire — Anecdotes. 2. Dogs — England
— Yorkshire — Biography. 3. Herriot, James. 4. Veterinarians —
England — Yorkshire — Biography. I. Title.
[SF426.2.H4725 1996b]
636.7—dc20   96-9023

Contents

James Herriot's Favorite
DOG STORIES

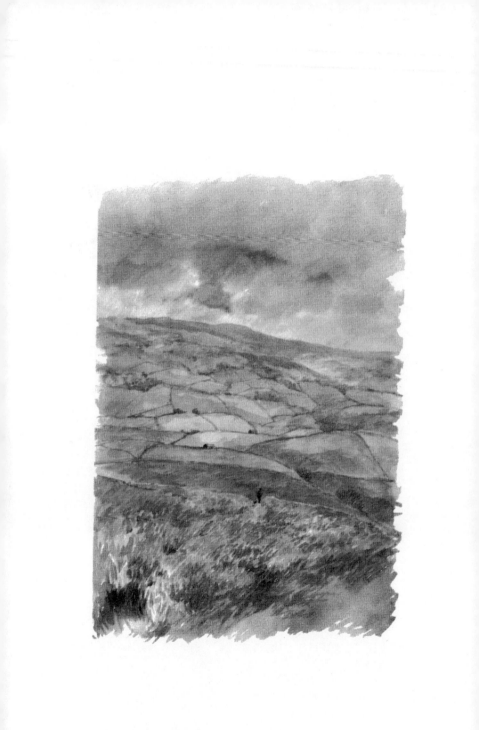

Introduction

"This was the real Yorkshire with the clean limestone wall riding the hill's edge and the path cutting brilliant green through the crowding heather. And, walking face on to the scented breeze, I felt the old tingle of wonder at being alone on the wide moorland where nothing stirred and the spreading miles of purple blossom and green turf reached away until it met the hazy blue of the sky."

Evocative stuff? Perhaps, but true. But what is truer still follows next in one of the stories included in this book:

"But I wasn't really alone. There

was Sam, and he made all the difference. Helen, my wife, had brought a lot of things into my life and Sam was one of the most precious. He was to be my faithful companion, my car dog, my friend who sat by my side through the lonely hours of driving. He was the first of a series of cherished dogs whose comradeship have warmed and lightened my working life" — and, latterly, my retirement.

Ever since I was a child, I have always loved dogs. Don, a beautiful sleek-coated Irish setter, was my first dog and I learned from an early age the pleasure that one gets from watching a dog — whether scenting after rabbits on the hillside, or indicating quite

Check Out Receipt

Newmarket Public Library

905-953-5110
www.newmarketpl.ca

Patron: SAUNDERS, CAROLYNN
Date: 12/21/2023 3:01:45 PM

1. **James Herriot's favorite dog stories**
   Barcode 35923001015173
   Due by 1/11/2024 11:59 PM

****

plainly that it is dinnertime, or sleeping in front of the fire, whiffling little noises, perhaps at the rabbits in his dreams.

When I decided I wanted to be a vet, I knew that I wanted to be a dog doctor, so I could spend all my time with dogs. But the authorities at the veterinary college in Glasgow had other ideas: at that time, in the mid-thirties, animals were graded according to their importance — horse, cattle, sheep, pig — and dog. And they decided I should be a horse doctor.

In due course, I qualified and was lucky to be offered a job as an assistant vet in North Yorkshire, in the town that I call Darrowby in my books. It was what is called a large-animal practice, the majority of patients being horses, cattle, sheep, and pigs. What chance was there of my becoming a dog doctor as I wanted? However, luck was on my side, because Siegfried Farnon, my boss (and later to be my partner) loved horses above everything else. He was more than happy to leave the dogs and cats to me while he attended to the Shire horses that were still being used at that time, and the hunters and ponies of the more affluent families.

As readers who know my books well will remember, I certainly did my fair share of work with the larger animals but I did love treating the smaller ones. Sometimes it was pure relief to be able to leave behind the cold, wet, and mud of the hillside and tend the ailments of some gentle little animal in a drawing room — and so you won't be surprised that I have included three stories in this book about the Peke Tricki Woo. Oh, that sherry — I can recall the taste of it now!

Driving out to the remote farms was a very lonely chore, especially during the winter, but one made a hundred times better when I had a dog or dogs with me in the car. Sam, my beagle — well, Helen's really — is mentioned several times in this book: he was very special and I can see him now, his big liquid eyes turned to me, suggesting we steal five minutes between appointments to walk on the high moors. I could rarely resist his plea — after all, I got so much pleasure too from standing for a while looking at the superb landscape spread out in front of me. There was everything here: wilderness and solitude breathing from the bare fells, yet a hint of softness where the river wound along the valley floor. And in all the green miles around me there was seldom another human being to be seen. I always had to force myself back into the real world when it was time to go, and when I called to Sam, he would come running up the track toward me, his ears flying in the wind, an almost human smile of contentment on his face.

After Sam, I had two dogs together. Hector was a Jack Russell with typical "Chippendale" legs and a stumpy tail which he wagged furiously. In the car he was never still; he would peer through the windscreen and seem to take in everything that we passed. My other dog, Dan the black Labrador, had a quite different temperament: he would stretch out on the passenger seat, his head on my knee, trusting that I wouldn't miss an opportunity to stop the car somewhere on the moor or in the dale and give them a run.

Dan is on the cover of my book *James Herriot's Yorkshire*: he was an old dog then — you can just see his graying muzzle against

15

the dark background of the trees in the snowy landscape behind. He is a little dipped in the back, but his eyes are fixed unwavering — not on me, but on the stick in my hand. Throughout his life, he liked to walk with a stick in his mouth, true retriever-fashion. As he got older, so the sticks he found to carry became smaller, and I knew that his life was coming to an end the day he returned from his walk without a stick. It is always said that however many wonderful and happy years a dog lives, you know that one day, the day he dies, your dog

16

will break your heart.

I have always advised people to get a replacement as soon as possible after their dog has died: a new and endearing pup helps enormously to fill the gaping void one always experiences after a much-loved dog has gone. But when Hector and Dan died, within a year of each other, but both having had good long lives, I hesitated: Would I ever be able to find a dog to replace them? I was still able to go on walks with a dog because my daughter Rosie, who lives next door to us, has a beautiful yellow Labrador, Polly, and was very happy that I wanted to take on dog-walking duties.

But the car was very empty

when I drove out to the farms or visited patients in outlying villages. When I got out to lean over a gate and look down into a valley, there was no one to watch snuffling amongst the heather and the bracken. There was no one to talk to — and the conversation may have been somewhat one-sided but my dogs never seemed to mind my chatter!

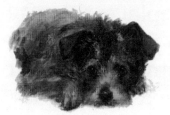 So I decided to fulfill a longtime ambition, to own a Border terrier. I had loved this breed, with its whiskery face, ever since I had come to work in Yorkshire, but there had never been a litter around when we had

wanted a new dog.

This time, however, I was very fortunate to find the last of a litter not far away in Bedale, and so Bodie joined the Herriot household. I don't think any of my other dogs would be too upset if I said that no dog has ever given me so much joy as Bodie — who is lying beside me now as I write. From the moment that I reached down and lifted up the puppy, and he curled his little body round, apparently trying to touch his tail with his nose, I was lost to him.

He has been a wonderful companion to me, especially since I retired and have had more time for walking. He is getting on now, and his coat is almost more white than brown; this has its advantages because I can see him when he is running through the autumn bracken when it is on the turn. When he was younger, he was almost the same color as the russety-red bracken and sometimes the only means I had of knowing where he had got to was by the high-pitched yelps emanating from the thick undergrowth, which meant that he was after another rabbit, which he very rarely caught. I know the chase gave him immense pleasure, however, because he would return to me, his tongue lolling out of the side of his mouth and a look on his face as if to say, "Well, there's always another day!"

He is a bit too old now to chase rabbits for real but he still whiffles in his sleep so I am sure he is chasing them in his dreams.

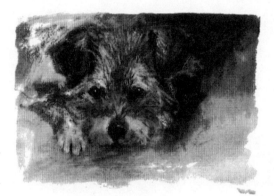

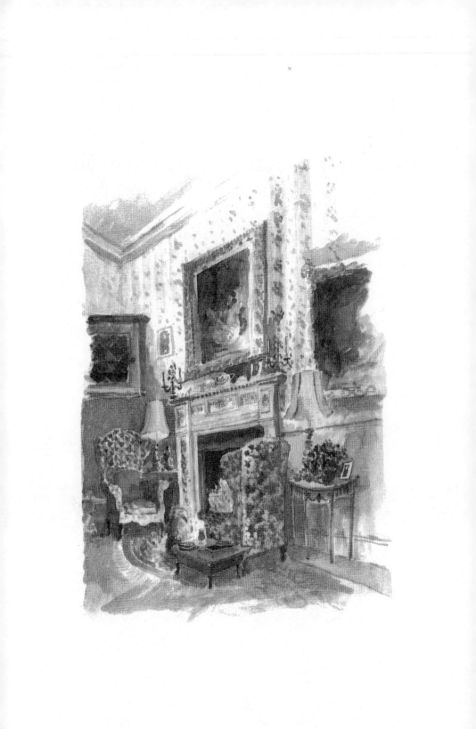

TRICKI WOO

Goes Crackerdog

Autumn had slipped into winter, the high tops were streaked with the first snows, and the discomforts of practice in the Dales began to make themselves felt.

Driving for hours with frozen feet, climbing to the high barns in biting winds which seared and flattened the wiry hill grass. The interminable stripping off in drafty buildings and the washing of hands and chest in buckets of cold water, using scrubbing soap and often a piece of sacking for a towel.

This was when some small animal work came as a blessed relief. To step out of the rough, hard routine for a while; to walk into a warm drawing room instead of a cow house and tackle something less formidable than a horse or a bull. And among all those comfortable drawing rooms there was none so beguiling as Mrs. Pumphrey's.

Mrs. Pumphrey was an elderly widow. Her late husband, a beer baron whose breweries and pubs were scattered widely over the broad bosom of Yorkshire, had left her a vast fortune and a beautiful house on the outskirts of Darrowby. Here she lived with a large staff of servants, a gardener, a chauffeur, and Tricki

Woo. Tricki Woo was a Pekingese and the apple of his mistress's eye.

Standing now in the magnificent doorway, I furtively rubbed the toes of my shoes on the backs of my trousers and blew on my cold hands. I could almost see the deep armchair drawn close to the leaping flames, the tray of cocktail biscuits, the bottle of excellent sherry. Because of the sherry, I was always careful to time my visits for half an hour before lunch.

A maid answered my ring, beaming on me as an honored guest, and led me to the room, crammed with expensive furniture and littered with glossy magazines and the latest novels.

Mrs. Pumphrey, in the high-backed chair by the fire, put down her book with a cry of delight. "Tricki! Tricki! Here is your Uncle Herriot!" I had been made an uncle very early and, sensing the advantages of the relationship, had made no objection.

Tricki, as always, bounded from his cushion, leaped onto the back of a sofa, and put his paws on my shoulders. He then licked my face thoroughly before retiring, exhausted. He was soon exhausted because he was given roughly twice the amount of food needed for a dog of his size. And it was the wrong kind of food.

"Oh, Mr. Herriot," Mrs. Pumphrey said, looking at her pet anxiously, "I'm so glad you've come. Tricki has gone flop-bott again."

This ailment, not to be found in any textbook, was her way of describing the symptoms of Tricki's impacted anal glands. When the glands filled up, he showed discomfort by sitting down suddenly in mid-walk and his mistress would rush to the phone in great agitation.

"Mr. Herriot, please come! He's going flop-bott again!"

I hoisted the little dog onto a table and very quickly sorted out his problem.

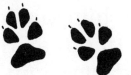

It baffled me that the Peke was always so pleased to see me. Any dog who could still like a man who grabbed him and squeezed his bottom hard every time they met had to have an incredibly forgiving nature. But Tricki never showed any resentment; in fact he was an outstandingly equable little animal, bursting with intelligence, and I was genuinely attached to him. It was a pleasure to be his personal physician.

The squeezing over, I lifted my patient from the table, noticing the increased weight, the padding of extra flesh over the ribs. "You know, Mrs. Pumphrey, you're overfeeding him again. Didn't I tell you to cut out all those pieces of cake and give him more protein?"

"Oh yes, Mr. Herriot," Mrs.

Pumphrey wailed. "But what can I do? He's so tired of chicken."

I shrugged; it was hopeless. I allowed the maid to lead me to the palatial bathroom so I could wash my hands. It was a huge room with a fully stocked dressing table, massive green jars, and rows of glass shelves laden with toilet preparations. My private guest towel was laid out next to the slab of expensive soap.

Then I returned to the drawing room, my sherry glass was filled, and I settled down by the fire to listen to Mrs. Pumphrey. It couldn't be called a conversation because she did all the talking, but I always found it rewarding.

Mrs. Pumphrey was likable, gave widely to charities, and

would help anybody in trouble. She was intelligent and amusing and had a lot of waffling charm; but most people have a blind spot and hers was Tricki Woo. The tales she told about her darling ranged far into the realms of fantasy and I waited eagerly for the next installment.

"Oh, Mr. Herriot, I have the most exciting news. Tricki has a pen pal! Yes, he wrote a letter to the editor of *Doggy World* enclosing a donation, and told him that even though he was descended from a long line of Chinese emperors, he had decided to come down and mingle freely with the common dogs. He asked the editor to seek out a pen pal for him among the dogs he knew so that they could correspond to their mutual benefit. And for this purpose, Tricki said he would adopt the name of Mr. Utterbunkum. And, do you know, he received the most beautiful letter from the editor" — I could imagine the sensible man leaping upon this potential gold mine — "who said he would like to introduce Bonzo Fotheringham, a lonely dalmatian who would be delighted to exchange letters with a new friend in Yorkshire."

I sipped the sherry. Tricki snored on my lap. Mrs. Pumphrey went on.

"But I'm so disappointed about the new summerhouse — you know I got it specially for Tricki so we could sit out together on warm afternoons. It's such a nice little rustic shelter, but he's taken a passionate dislike to it. Simply loathes it — absolutely

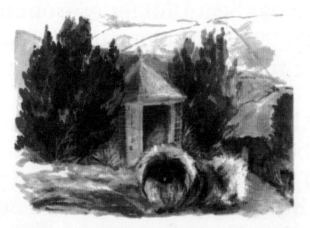

refuses to go inside. You should see the dreadful expression on his face when he looks at it. And do you know what he called it yesterday? Oh, I hardly dare tell you." She looked around the room before leaning over and whispering: "He called it 'the bloody hut'!"

The maid struck fresh life into the fire and refilled my glass. The wind hurled a handful of sleet against the window. This, I thought, was the life. I listened for more.

"And did I tell you, Mr. Herriot, Tricki had another good win yesterday? You know, I'm sure he must study the racing columns, he's such a tremendous judge of form. Well, he told me to back Canny Lad in the three o'clock at Redcar yesterday and, as usual, it won. He put on a shilling each way and got back nine shillings."

These bets were always placed in the name of Tricki Woo and I thought with compassion of the reactions of the local bookies. The Darrowby turf accountants were a harassed and fugitive body of men. A board would appear at the end of some alley urging the population to invest with Joe Downs and enjoy perfect security. Joe would live for a few months on a knife edge while he pitted his wits against the knowledge-able citizens, but the end was always the same; a few favorites would win in a row and Joe would be gone in the night, tak-ing his board with him. Once I had asked a local inhabitant about the sudden departure of one of these luckless nomads. He replied unemotionally, "Oh, we broke him. He won't be back in a hurry."

Losing a regular flow of shillings to a dog must have been a heavy cross for these unfortunate men to bear.

"I had such a frightening experience last week," Mrs. Pumphrey continued. "I was sure I would have to call you out. Poor little Tricki — he went completely crackerdog!"

I mentally lined this up with flop-bott among the new canine diseases and asked for more information.

"It was awful. I was terrified. The gardener was throwing rings for Tricki — you know he does this for half an hour every day." I had witnessed this spectacle several times. Hodgkin, a dour, bent old Yorkshireman who looked as though he hated all dogs and Tricki in particular, had to go out on the lawn every day and throw little rubber rings over and over again. Tricki bounded after them and brought them back, barking madly until the process was repeated. The bitter lines on the old man's face deepened as the game progressed. His lips moved continually, but it was impossible to hear what he was saying.

Mrs. Pumphrey went on: "Well, he was playing his game, and he does adore it so, when suddenly, without warning, he went crackerdog. He forgot about his rings and began to run around in circles, barking and yelping in such a strange way. Then he fell over

36

on his side and lay like a little dead thing. Do you know, Mr. Herriot, I really thought he was dead, he lay so perfectly still. And what hurt me most was that Hodgkin began to laugh. He has been with me for twenty-four years and I have never ever seen him smile, and yet, when he looked down at that still form, he broke into a queer, high-pitched cackle. It was horrid. I was just going to rush to the telephone when Tricki got up and walked away — he seemed perfectly normal."

Hysteria, I thought, brought on by wrong feeding and overexcitement. I put down my glass and fixed Mrs. Pumphrey with a severe glare. "Now look, this is just what I was talking about. If you persist in feeding all that fancy rubbish to Tricki you are going to ruin his health. You really must get him on to a sensible dog diet of one, or at the most, two small meals a day of meat and brown bread or a little biscuit. And nothing in between."

Mrs. Pumphrey shrank into her chair, a picture of abject guilt. "Oh, please don't speak to me like that. I do try to give him the right things, but it is so difficult. When he begs for his little tidbits, I can't refuse him." She dabbed her eyes with a handkerchief.

But I was unrelenting. "All right, Mrs. Pumphrey, it's up to you, but I warn you that if you go on as you are doing, Tricki will go crackerdog more and more often."

I left the cozy haven with reluctance, pausing on the graveled drive to look back at Mrs. Pumphrey waving and Tricki, as always, standing against the window, his wide-mouthed face apparently in the middle of a hearty laugh.

Driving home, I mused on the many advantages of being Tricki's uncle. When he went to the seaside he sent me boxes of oak-smoked kippers; and when the tomatoes ripened in his greenhouse, he sent a pound or two every week. Tins of tobacco arrived regularly, sometimes with a photograph carrying a loving inscription.

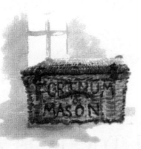

But it was when the Christmas hamper arrived from Fortnum & Mason's that I decided that I was on a really good thing which should be helped along a bit. Hitherto, I had merely run up and thanked Mrs. Pumphrey for the gifts, and she had been rather cool, pointing out that it was Tricki who had sent the things and he was the one who should be thanked.

With the arrival of the hamper it came to me, blindingly, that I had been guilty of a grave error of tactics. I set myself to compose a letter to Tricki. Avoiding my partner Siegfried's sardonic eye,

I thanked my doggy nephew for his Christmas gifts and for all his generosity in the past. I expressed my sincere hopes that the festive fare had not upset his delicate digestion and suggested that if he did experience any discomfort he should have recourse to the black powder his uncle always prescribed. A vague feeling of professional shame was easily swamped by floating visions of kippers, tomatoes, and hampers. I addressed the envelope to Master Tricki Pumphrey, Barlby Grange, and slipped it into the post with only a slight feeling of guilt.

On my next visit, Mrs. Pumphrey drew me to one side. "Mr. Herriot," she whispered, "Tricki adored your charming letter and he will keep it always, but he was very put out about one thing — you addressed it to Master Tricki and he does insist upon Mister. He was dreadfully affronted at first, quite beside himself, but when he saw it was from you he soon recovered his good temper. I can't think why he should have these little prejudices. Perhaps it is because he is an only dog — I do think an only dog develops more prejudices than one from a larger family."

Entering Skeldale House was like returning to a colder world. Siegfried bumped into me in the passage. "Ah, who have we here? Why I do believe it's dear Uncle Herriot. And what have you been doing, Uncle? Slaving away at Barlby Grange, I expect. Poor fellow, you must be tired out. Do you really think it's worth it, working your fingers to the bone for another hamper?"

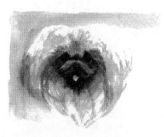

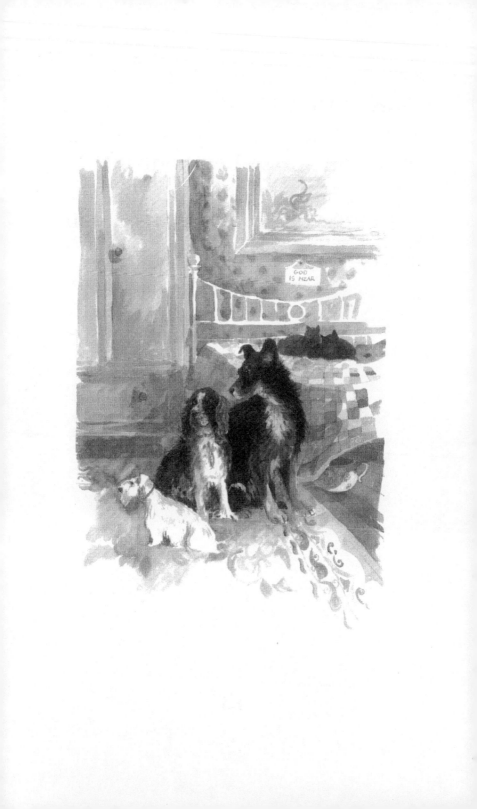

PRINCE

and the Card Above the Bed

The card dangled above the old lady's bed. It read GOD IS NEAR but it wasn't like the usual religious text. It didn't have a frame or ornate printing. It was just a strip of cardboard about eight inches long with plain lettering which might have said "No smoking" or "Exit" and it was looped carelessly over an old brass gas bracket so that Miss Stubbs from where she lay could look up at it and read GOD IS NEAR in square black capitals.

There wasn't much more Miss

Stubbs could see; perhaps a few feet of privet hedge through the frayed curtains but mainly it was just the cluttered little room which had been her world for so many years.

The room was on the ground floor and in the front of the cottage, and as I came up through

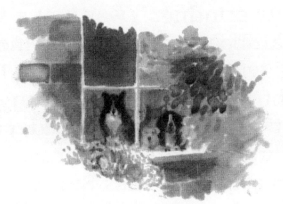

the wilderness which had once been a garden I could see the dogs watching me from where they had jumped onto the old lady's bed by the window. And when I knocked on the door the place almost erupted with their barking. It was always like this. I had been visiting regularly for over a year and the pattern never changed; the furious barking, then Mrs. Broadwith, who looked after Miss Stubbs, would push all the animals but my patient into the back kitchen and open the door and I would go in and see Miss Stubbs in the corner in her bed with the card hanging over it.

She had been there for a long time and would never get up again. But she never mentioned her illness and pain to me; all her concern was for her three dogs and two cats.

Today it was old Prince and I was worried about him. It was his heart — just about the most spectacular valvular incompetence I had ever heard. He was waiting for me as I came in, pleased to see me, his long fringed tail waving gently.

The sight of that tail used to make me think there must be a lot of Irish setter in Prince but I was inclined to change my mind as I worked my way forward over the bulging black and brown body to the shaggy head and up-standing Alsatian-type ears — well, at least he kept one of them upright but the other tipped over at the top. Miss Stubbs often used to call him "Mr. Heinz" and though he may not have had 57 varieties in him, his hybrid vigor had stood him in good stead. With his heart he should have been dead long ago.

"I thought I'd best give you a ring, Mr. Herriot," Mrs. Broadwith said. She was a comfortable, elderly widow with a square, ruddy face contrasting sharply with the pinched features on the pillow. "He's been coughing right bad this week and this morning he was a bit staggery. Still eats well, though."

"I bet he does." I ran my hands over the rolls of fat on the ribs. "It would take something really drastic to put old Prince off his grub."

Miss Stubbs laughed from the bed and the old dog, his mouth

wide, eyes dancing, seemed to be joining in the joke. I put my stethoscope over his heart and listened, knowing well what I was going to hear. They say the heart is supposed to go "Lub-dup, lub-dup," but Prince's went "swish-swoosh, swish-swoosh." There seemed to be nearly as much blood leaking back as was being pumped into the circulatory system. And another thing, the "swish-swoosh" was a good bit faster than last time; he was on oral digitalis but it wasn't quite doing its job.

Gloomily I moved the stethoscope over the rest of the chest. Like all old dogs with a chronic heart weakness he had an ever-present bronchitis and I listened without enthusiasm to the symphony of whistles, babbles, squeaks and bubbles which signaled the workings of Prince's lungs. The old dog stood very erect and proud, his tail still waving slowly. He always took it as a tremendous compliment when I examined him and there was no doubt he was enjoying himself now. Fortunately his was not a very painful ailment.

Straightening up, I patted his head, and he responded immediately by trying to put his paws on my chest. He didn't quite make it and even that slight exertion started his ribs heaving and his tongue lolling. I gave him an intramuscular injection of digitalin and another of morphine hydrochloride, which he accepted with apparent pleasure as part of the game.

"I hope that will steady his heart and breathing, Miss Stubbs. You'll find he'll be a bit dopey for the rest of the day and that will help, too. Carry on with the tablets as before, and I'm going to leave you some more medicine for his bronchitis."

The next stage of the visit began now as Mrs. Broadwith brought in a cup of tea and the rest of the animals were let out of the kitchen. There were Ben, a Sealyham, and Sally, a cocker spaniel, and they started a deafening barking contest with Prince. They were closely followed by the cats, Arthur and Susie, who stalked in gracefully and began to rub themselves against my trouser legs.

It was the usual scenario for the many cups of tea I had drunk with Miss Stubbs under the little card which dangled above her bed.

"How are you today?" I asked.

"Oh, much better," she replied and immediately, as always, changed the subject.

Mostly she liked to talk about her pets and the ones she had known right back to her girlhood. She spoke a lot, too, about the days when her family were alive. She loved to describe the escapades of her three brothers and today she showed me a photograph which Mrs. Broadwith had found at the bottom of a drawer.

I took it from her and three young men in the knee breeches and little round caps of the eighteen-nineties smiled up at me from the yellowed old print; they all held long church warden pipes and the impish humor in their expressions came down undimmed over the years.

"My word, they look really bright lads, Miss Stubbs," I said.

"Oh, they were young rips!" she exclaimed. She threw back her head and laughed and for a moment her face was radiant, transfigured by her memories.

The things I had heard in the village came back to me; about the prosperous father and his family who lived in the big house many years ago. Then the foreign investments which crashed and the sudden change in circumstances. "When t'owd feller died he was about skint," one old man had said. "There's not much brass there now."

Probably just enough brass to keep Miss Stubbs and her animals alive and to pay Mrs. Broadwith. Not enough to keep the garden dug or the house painted or for any of the normal little luxuries.

And, sitting there, drinking my tea, with the dogs in a row by the bedside and the cats making themselves comfortable on the bed itself, I felt as I had often felt before — a bit afraid of the responsibility I had. The one thing which brought some light into the life of the brave old woman was the transparent devotion of this shaggy bunch whose eyes were never far from her face. And the snag was that they were all elderly.

There had, in fact, been four dogs originally, but one of them, a truly ancient yellow Labrador, had died a few months previously. And now I had the rest of them to look after and none of them less than ten years old.

They were perky enough but all showing some of the signs of old age; Prince with his heart, Sally beginning to drink a lot of water which made me wonder if her kidneys were giving trouble; Ben growing steadily thinner with his nephritis. I couldn't give him new kidneys and I hadn't much faith in the tablets I had prescribed. Another peculiar thing about Ben was that I was always having to clip his claws; they grew at an extraordinary rate.

The cats were better, though Susie was a bit scraggy and I kept up a morbid kneading of her furry abdomen for signs of lymphosarcoma. Arthur was the best of the bunch; he never seemed to ail anything beyond a tendency for his teeth to attract tartar.

This must have been in Miss Stubbs's mind because, when I had finished my tea, she asked me to look at him. I hauled him across the bedspread and opened his mouth.

"Yes, there's a bit of the old trouble there. Might as well fix it while I'm here."

Arthur was a huge, gray neutered tom, a living denial of all those theories that cats are cold-natured, selfish, and the rest. His fine eyes, framed in the widest cat face I have ever seen, looked out on the world with an all-embracing benevolence and tolerance. His every movement was marked by immense dignity.

As I started to scrape his teeth his chest echoed with a booming purr like a distant outboard motor. There was no need for anybody to hold him; he sat there placidly and moved only once — when I was using forceps to crack off a tough piece of tartar from a back tooth and accidentally nicked his gum. He casually raised a massive paw as if to say "Have a care, chum," but his claws were sheathed.

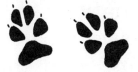

My next visit was less than a month later and was in response to an urgent summons from Mrs. Broadwith at six o'clock in the evening. Ben had collapsed. I jumped straight into my car and in less than ten minutes was threading my way through the overgrown grass in the front garden with just two dogs watching from their window. The barking broke out as I knocked, but Ben's was absent. As I went into the little room I saw the old dog lying on his side, very still, by the bed.

D.O.A. is what we write in the day book. Dead On Arrival. Just three words but they covered all kinds of situations — the end of milk fever cows, bloated bullocks, calves in fits. And tonight they meant that I wouldn't be clipping old Ben's claws anymore.

"Well, it was quick, Miss Stubbs. I'm sure the old chap didn't suffer at all." My words sounded lame and ineffectual.

The old lady was in full command of herself. No tears, only a fixity of expression as she looked down from the bed at her companion for so many years. My idea was to get him out of the place as quickly as possible and

I pulled a blanket under him and lifted him up. As I was moving away, Miss Stubbs said, "Wait a moment." With an effort she turned on her side and gazed at Ben. Still without changing expression, she reached out and touched his head lightly. Then she lay back calmly as I hurried from the room.

In the back kitchen I had a whispered conference with Mrs. Broadwith. "I'll run down t'village and get Fred Manners to come and bury him," she said. "And if you've got time, could you stay with the old lady while I'm gone. Talk to her, like, it'll do her good."

I went back and sat down by the bed. Miss Stubbs looked out of the window for a few moments, then turned to me. "You know, Mr. Herriot," she said casually, "it will be my turn next."

"What do you mean?"

"Well, tonight Ben has gone and I'm going to be the next one. I just know it."

"Oh, nonsense! You're feeling a bit low, that's all. We all do when something like this happens." But I was disturbed. I had never heard her even hint at such a thing before.

"I'm not afraid," she said. "I know there's something better waiting for me. I've never had any doubts." There was silence between us as she lay calmly looking up at the card on the gas bracket.

Then the head on the pillow

turned to me again. "I have only one fear." Her expression changed with startling suddenness as if a mask had dropped. The brave face was almost unrecognizable. A kind of terror flickered in her eyes and she quickly grasped my hand.

"It's the dogs and cats, Mr. Herriot. I'm afraid I might never see them when I'm gone which worries me so. You see, I know I'll be reunited with my parents and brothers, but . . . but . . ." She gazed at the two cats curled up at the end of her bed.

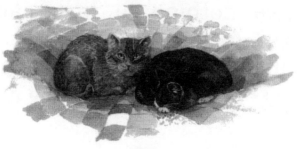

"Well, why not with your animals?"

"That's just it." She rocked her head on the pillow and for the first time I saw tears on her cheeks. "They say animals have no souls."

"Who says?"

"Oh, I've read it and I know a lot of religious people believe it."

"Well, I don't believe it." I patted the hand which still grasped mine. "If having a soul means being able to feel love and loyalty and gratitude, then animals are better off than a lot of humans. You've nothing to worry about there."

"Oh, I hope you're right. Sometimes I lie at night thinking about it."

64

"I know I'm right, Miss Stubbs, and don't you argue with me. They teach us vets all about animals' souls."

The tension left her face and she laughed with a return of her old spirit. "I'm sorry to bore you with this and I'm not going to talk about it again. But before you go, I want you to be absolutely honest with me. I don't want reassurance from you — just the truth. I know you are very young but please tell me — what are your beliefs? Will my animals go with me?"

She stared intently into my eyes. I shifted in my chair and swallowed once or twice.

"Miss Stubbs, I'm afraid I'm a bit foggy about all this," I said.

"But I'm absolutely certain of one thing. Wherever you are going, they are going too."

She still stared at me but her face was calm again. "Thank you, Mr. Herriot, I know you are being honest with me. That is what you really believe, isn't it?"

"I do believe it," I said. "With all my heart I believe it."

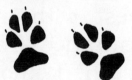

It must have been about a month later and it was entirely by accident that I learned I had seen Miss Stubbs for the last time. When a lonely, penniless old woman dies people don't rush up to you in the street to tell you. I was on my rounds and a farmer happened to mention that the cottage in Corby village was up for sale.

"But what about Miss Stubbs?" I asked.

"Oh, went off sudden about three weeks ago. House is in a bad state, they say — nowt been done at it for years."

"Mrs. Broadwith isn't staying on, then?"

"Nay, I hear she's staying at t'other end of village."

"Do you know what's happened to the dogs and cats?"

"What dogs and cats?"

I cut my visit short. And I didn't go straight home, though it was nearly lunchtime. Instead I urged my complaining little car at top speed to Corby and asked the first person I saw where Mrs. Broadwith was living. It was a tiny house but attractive and Mrs. Broadwith answered my knock herself.

"Oh, come in, Mr. Herriot. It's right good of you to call." I went inside and we sat facing each other across a scrubbed tabletop.

"Well, it was sad about the old lady," she said.

"Yes, I've only just heard."

"Any road, she had a peaceful end. Just slept away at finish."

"I'm glad to hear that."

Mrs. Broadwith looked round the room. "I was real lucky to get this place — it's just what I've always wanted."

I could contain myself no longer. "What's happened to the

animals?" I blurted out.

"Oh, they're in t'garden," she said calmly. "I've got a grand big stretch at back." She got up and opened the door and with a surge of relief I watched my old friends pour in.

Arthur was on my knee in a flash, arching himself ecstatically against my arm while his out-board motor roared softly above the barking of the dogs. Prince, wheezy as ever, tail fanning the air, laughed up at me delightedly between barks.

"They look great, Mrs. Broad-with. How long are they going to be here?"

"They're here for good. I think just as much about them as t'old lady ever did and I couldn't be parted from them. They'll have a good home with me as long as they live."

I looked at the typical Yorkshire country face, at the heavy cheeks with their grim lines belied by the kindly eyes. "This is wonderful," I said. "But won't you find it just a bit . . . er . . . expensive to feed them?"

"Nay, you don't have to worry about that. I 'ave a bit put away."

"Well, fine, fine, and I'll be looking in now and then to see how they are. I'm through the village every few days." I got up and started for the door.

Mrs. Broadwith held up her hand. "There's just one thing I'd like you to do before they start selling off the things at the cottage. Would you please pop in and collect what's left of your medicines. They're in t'front room."

I took the key and drove along to the other end of the village. As I pushed open the rickety gate and began to walk through the tangled grass, the front of the cottage looked strangely lifeless without the faces of the dogs at the window; and when the door creaked open and I went inside the silence was like a heavy pall.

Nothing had been moved. The bed with its rumpled blankets was still in the corner. I moved around, picking up half-empty bottles, a jar of ointment, the cardboard box with old Ben's tablets — a lot of good they had done him.

When I had got everything I looked slowly round the little room. I wouldn't be coming here anymore and at the door I paused and read for the last time the card which hung over the empty bed.

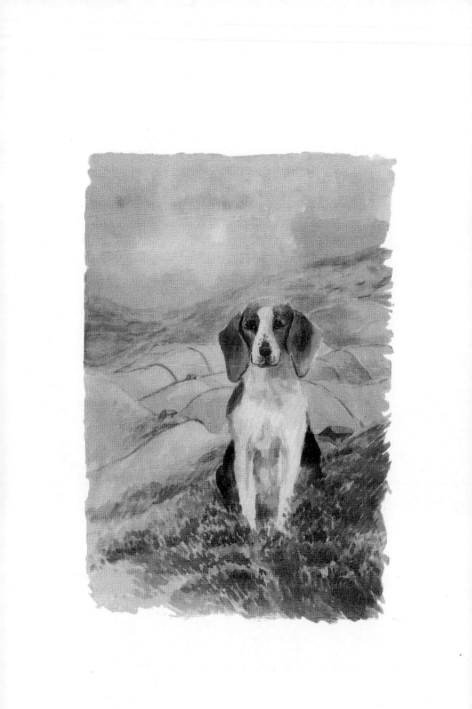

JOCK

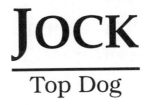

Top Dog

I had only to sit up in bed to look right across Darrowby to the hills beyond.

I got up and walked to the window. It was going to be a fine morning and the early sun glanced over the weathered reds and grays of the jumbled roofs, some of them sagging under their burden of ancient tiles, and brightened the tufts of green where trees pushed upward from the gardens among the bristle of chimney pots. And behind everything the calm bulk of the fells.

It was my good fortune that this was the first thing I saw every morning; after Helen, of course, which was better still.

Following our honeymoon we had set up our first home in the top of Skeldale House. Siegfried, my boss up to my wedding and now my partner, had offered us free use of these empty rooms on the third story and we had gratefully accepted; and though it was a makeshift arrangement there was an airy charm, an exhilaration in our high perch that many would have envied.

Helen soon had the kettle boiling and we drank our first cup of tea by the window looking down on the long garden. From up here we had an aerial view of the unkept lawns, the fruit trees, the wisteria climbing the weathered brick toward our window, and the high walls with their old stone copings stretching away to the cobbled yard under the elms. Every day I went up and down that path to the garage in the yard but it looked so different from above.

After breakfast I went downstairs, collected my gear, including suture material for a foal which had cut its leg, and went out the side door into the garden. Just about opposite the rockery I turned and looked up at our window. It was open at the bottom and an arm emerged holding a dishcloth. I waved and the dishcloth waved back furiously. It was the start to every day.

And, driving from the yard, it seemed a good start. In fact everything was good. The raucous cawing of the rooks in the trees above, the clean fragrance of the air which greeted me every morning, and the challenge and interest of my job.

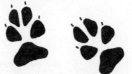

This was the real Yorkshire with the clean limestone wall riding the hill's edge and the path cutting brilliant green through the crowding heather. And, walking face on to the scented breeze, I felt the old tingle of wonder at being alone on the wide moorland where nothing stirred and the spreading miles of purple blossom and green turf reached away until it met the hazy blue of the sky.

But I wasn't really alone. There was Sam, and he made all the difference. Helen had brought a lot of things into my life and Sam was one of the most precious; he was a beagle and her own personal pet. He would have been about two years old when I first saw him and I had no way of knowing that he was to be my faithful companion, my car dog, my friend who sat by my side through the lonely hours of driving until his life ended at the age of fourteen. He was the first of a series of cherished dogs whose comradeship have warmed and lightened my working life.

Sam adopted me on sight. It was as though he had read the *Faithful Hound Manual* because he was always near me; paws on the dashboard, as he gazed eagerly through the windscreen on my rounds, head resting on my foot in our bed-sitting room, trotting just behind me wherever I moved. If I had a beer in a pub he would be under my chair and even when I was having a haircut you only had to lift the white sheet to see Sam crouching beneath my legs. The only place I didn't dare take him was to the cinema and on these occasions he crawled under the bed and sulked.

Most dogs love car riding but to

Sam it was a passion which never waned — even in the night hours; he would gladly leave his basket when the world was asleep, stretch a couple of times and follow me out into the cold. He would be onto the seat before I got the car door fully open and this action became so much a part of my life that for a long time after his death I still held the door open unthinkingly, waiting for him. And I still remember the pain I felt when he did not bound inside.

And having him with me added so much to the intermissions I granted myself on my daily rounds. Whereas in offices and factories they had tea breaks I just stopped the car and stepped out into the splendor which was always at hand and walked for a spell down hidden lanes, through woods, or, as today, along one of the grassy tracks which ran over the high tops. I like my fellow men but there are times when it is wonderful to be utterly alone in a wide landscape. Here I can find peace and tranquility.

This thing which I had always done had a new meaning now. Anybody who has ever walked a dog knows the abiding satisfaction which comes from giving pleasure to a loved animal, and the sight of the little form trotting ahead of me lent a depth which had been missing before.

The dry stone walls climbed up the bare hillsides on the far side of the valley. Those wonderful walls, often the only sign of the hand of man, symbolize the very soul of the high Pennines, the endlessly varying pattern of gray against green, carving out ragged squares and oblongs, pushing long antennae to impossible heights until they disappear into the lapping moorland on the summits.

Round the curve of the path I came to where the tide of heather lapped thickly down the hillside on a little slope facing invitingly into the sun. It was a call I could never resist. I looked at my watch; oh, I had a few minutes to spare before my appointment with Robert Corner. In a moment I was stretched out on the springy stems, the most wonderful natural mattress in the world.

Lying there, eyes half closed against the sun's glare, the heavy heather fragrance around me, I could see the cloud shadows racing across the flanks of the fells, throwing the gulleys and crevices into momentary gloom but trailing a fresh flaring green in their wake.

Those were the days when I was most grateful I was in country practice; the shirtsleeve days when the bleak menace of the bald heights melted into friendliness, when I felt at one with all the airy life and growth about me and was glad that I had become what I never thought I would be, a doctor of farm animals.

A long-eared head blotted out the sunshine as Sam came and sat on my chest. He looked at me questioningly. He didn't hold with this laziness but I knew if I didn't move after a few minutes he would curl up philosophically on my ribs and have a sleep until I was ready to go. But this time I answered the unspoken appeal by sitting up and he leaped around me in delight as I rose and began to make my way back to the car.

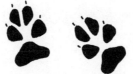

The injured foal was at Robert Corner's farm and I hadn't been there long before I spotted Jock, his sheepdog. And I began to watch the dog because behind a vet's daily chore at treating his patients there is always the fascinating kaleidoscope of animal personality and Jock was an interesting case.

A lot of farm dogs are partial to a little light relief from their work. They like to play and one of their favorite games is chasing cars off the premises. Often I drove off with a hairy form galloping alongside and the dog would usually give a final defiant bark after a few hundred yards to speed me on my way. But Jock was different.

He was really dedicated. Car chasing to him was a deadly serious art which he practiced daily without a trace of levity. Corner's farm was at the end of a long track, twisting for nearly a mile between its stone walls down through the gently sloping fields to the road below, and Jock didn't consider he had done his job properly until he had escorted his chosen vehicle right to the very foot. So his hobby was an exacting one.

I watched him now as I finished stitching the foal's leg and began to tie on a bandage. He was slinking about the buildings, a skinny little creature who without his mass of black and white hair would have been an almost invisible mite, and he was playing out a transparent charade of pretending he was taking no notice of me — wasn't the least bit interested in my presence, in fact. But his furtive glances in the direction of the stable, his repeated crisscrossing of my line of vision, gave him away. He was waiting for his big moment.

When I was putting on my shoes and throwing my wellingtons into the trunk, I saw him again. Or rather part of him; just a long nose and one eye protruding from beneath a broken door. It wasn't until I had started the engine and begun to

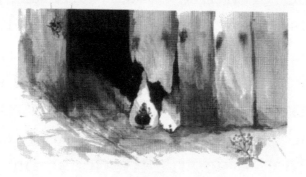

move off that he finally declared himself, stealing out from his hiding place, body low, tail trailing, eyes fixed intently on the car's front wheels, and as I gathered speed and headed down the track he broke into an effortless lope.

I had been through this before and was always afraid he might run in front of me so I put my foot down and began to hurtle downhill. This was where Jock came into his own. I often wondered how he'd fare against a racing greyhound because by golly he could run. That sparse frame housed a perfect physical machine and the slender limbs reached and flew again and again, devouring the stony ground beneath, keeping up with the speeding car with joyful ease.

There is a sharp bend about halfway down and here Jock invariably sailed over the wall and streaked across the turf, a little dark blur against the green, and having craftily cut off the corner he reappeared again like a missile zooming over the gray stones lower down. This put him into a nice position for the run to the road and when he finally saw me onto the tarmac my last view of him was of a happy panting face looking after me. Clearly he considered it was a job well done and he would wander contentedly back up to the farm to await the next exciting session, perhaps with the postman or the baker's van.

And there was another side to Jock. He was an outstanding performer at the sheepdog trials and Mr. Corner had won many trophies with him. In fact the farmer could have sold the little animal for a lot of money but couldn't be persuaded to part with him. Instead he purchased a bitch, a scrawny little female counterpart of Jock and a trial winner in her own right. With this combination Mr. Corner thought he could breed some world-beating types for sale. On my visits to the farm the bitch joined in the car-chasing but it seemed as though she was doing it more or less to humor her new mate and she always gave up at the first bend, leaving Jock in command. You could see her heart wasn't in it.

Then the pups arrived, seven fluffy black-and-white balls tumbling about the yard and getting under everybody's feet. Jock watched indulgently as they tried to follow him in his pursuit of my vehicle and you could almost see him laughing as they fell over their feet and were left trailing far behind.

It happened that I didn't have to go there for about ten months but I saw Robert Corner in the market occasionally and he told me he was training the pups and they were shaping well. Not that they needed much training; it was in their blood and he said they had tried to round up the cattle and sheep nearly as soon as they could walk. When I finally saw them they were like seven Jocks — meager, darting little creatures flitting noiselessly about the buildings — and it didn't

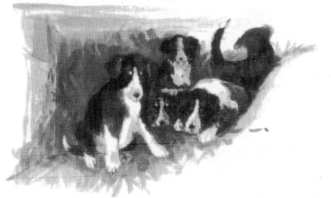

take me long to find out that they had learned more than sheep herding from their father. There was something very evocative about the way they began to prowl around in the background as I prepared to get into my car, peeping furtively from behind straw bales, slinking with elaborate nonchalance into favorable positions for a quick getaway. And as I settled in my seat I could sense they were all crouched in readiness for the off.

I revved my engine, let in the clutch with a bump and shot across the yard and in a second the immediate vicinity erupted in a mass of hairy forms. I roared onto the track and put my foot down and on either side of me the little animals pelted along shoulder to shoulder, their faces all wearing the intent fanatical expression I knew so well. When Jock cleared the wall the seven pups went with him and when they reappeared and entered the home straight I noticed something different. On past occasions Jock had always had one eye on the car — this was what he considered his opponent; but now on that last quarter mile as he hurtled along at the head of a shaggy phalanx he was glancing at the pups on either side as though they were the main opposition.

And there was no doubt he was in trouble. Superbly fit though he was, these stringy bundles of bone and sinew which he had fathered had all his speed plus the newly minted energy of youth. It was taking every shred of his power to keep up with them. Indeed there was one terrible moment when he stumbled and was engulfed by the bounding creatures around him; it seemed that all was lost, but there was a core of steel in Jock. Eyes popping, nostrils dilated, he fought his way through the pack until by the time we reached the road he was once more in the lead.

But it had taken its toll. I slowed down before driving away and looked down at the little animal standing with lolling tongue and heaving flanks on the grass verge. It must have been like this with all the other vehicles and it wasn't a merry game anymore. I suppose it sounds silly to say you could read a dog's thoughts, but everything in his posture betrayed the mounting apprehension that his days of supremacy were numbered. Just round the

corner lay the unthinkable igno-
miny of being left trailing in the
rear of that litter of young up-
starts, and as I drew away Jock
looked after me and his expression was eloquent.

"How long can I keep this up?"

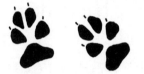

I felt for the little dog and on
my next visit to the farm about
two months later I wasn't looking
forward to witnessing the final
degradation which I felt was inevitable. But when I drove into
the yard I found the place
strangely unpopulated.

Robert Corner was forking hay
into the cows' racks in the byre.
He turned as I came in.

"Where are all your dogs?" I asked.

He put down his fork. "All gone. By gaw, there's a market for good workin' sheepdogs. I've done right well out of t'job."

"But you've still got Jock?"

"Oh, aye, ah couldn't part with t'awd lad. He's over there."

And so he was, creeping around as of old, pretending he wasn't watching me. And when the happy time finally arrived and I drove away it was like it used to be with the lean little animal haring along by the side of the car, but relaxed, enjoying the game, winging effortlessly over the wall and beating the car down to the tarmac with no trouble at all.

I think I was as relieved as he

was that he was left alone with his supremacy unchallenged; that he was still top dog.

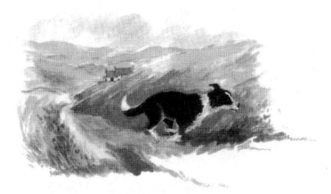

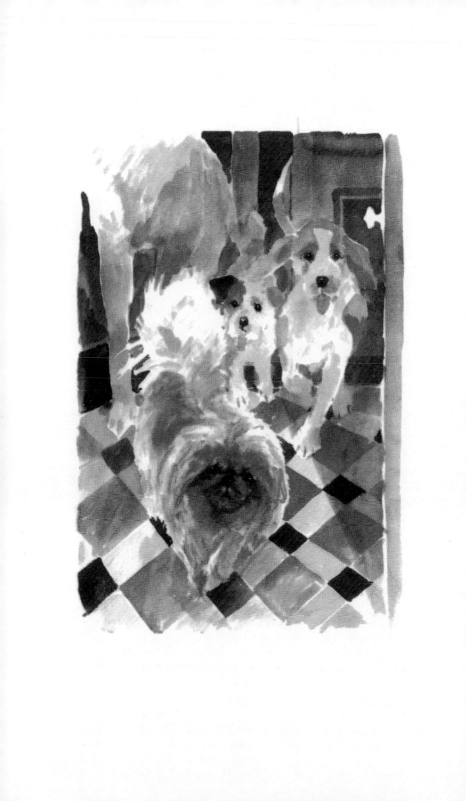

TRICKI WOO

A Triumph of Surgery

I was really worried about Tricki this time. I had pulled up my car when I saw him in the street with his mistress and I was shocked at his appearance. He had become hugely fat, like a bloated sausage with a leg at each corner. His eyes, bloodshot and rheumy, stared straight ahead, and his tongue lolled from his jaws.

Mrs. Pumphrey hastened to explain. "He was so listless, Mr. Herriot. He seemed to have no energy. I thought he must be suffering from malnutrition, so I have been giving him some little extras between meals to build him up. Some calf's foot jelly and malt and cod liver oil and a bowl of Horlick's at night to make him sleep — nothing much really."

"And did you cut down on the sweet things as I told you?"

"Oh, I did for a bit, but he seemed to be so weak. I had to relent. He does love cream cakes and chocolates so. I can't bear to refuse him."

I looked down again at the little dog. That was the trouble. Tricki's only fault was greed. He had never been known to refuse food; he would tackle a meal at any hour of the day or night. And I wondered about all the things Mrs. Pumphrey hadn't mentioned, the pâté on thin biscuits, the fudge, the rich trifles — Tricki loved them all.

"Are you giving him plenty of exercise?"

"Well, he has his little walks with me as you can see, but Hodgkin has been down with lumbago, so there has been no ring-throwing lately."

I tried to sound severe. "Now I really mean this. If you don't cut his food right down and give him more exercise he is going to be really ill. You must harden your heart and keep him on a very strict diet."

Mrs. Pumphrey wrung her hands. "Oh, I will, Mr. Herriot. I'm sure you are right, but it is so difficult, so very difficult." She set off, head down, along the road, as if determined to put the new régime into practice immediately.

I watched their progress with growing concern. Tricki was tottering along in his little tweed coat; he had a whole wardrobe of these coats — warm tweed or tartan ones for the cold weather and mackintoshes for the wet days. He struggled on, drooping in his harness. I thought it wouldn't be long before I heard from Mrs. Pumphrey.

The expected call came within a few days. Mrs. Pumphrey was distraught. Tricki would eat nothing. Refused even his favorite dishes; and besides, he had bouts of vomiting. He spent all his time lying on a rug, panting.

Didn't want to go on walks, didn't want to do anything.

I had made my plans in advance. The only way was to get Tricki out of the house for a period. I suggested that he be hospitalized for about a fortnight to be kept under observation.

The poor lady almost swooned. She had never been separated from her darling before; she was sure he would pine and die if he did not see her every day.

But I took a firm line. Tricki was very ill and this was the only way to save him; in fact, I thought it best to take him without delay and, followed by Mrs. Pumphrey's wailings, I marched out to the car carrying the little dog wrapped in a blanket.

The entire staff was roused and maids rushed in and out bringing his day bed, his night bed, favorite cushions, toys and rubber rings, breakfast bowl, lunch bowl, supper bowl. Realizing that

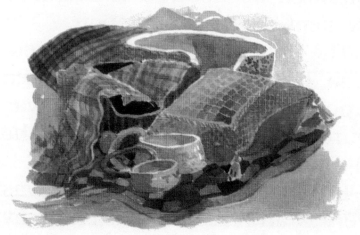

my car would never hold all the stuff, I started to drive away. As I moved off, Mrs. Pumphrey, with a despairing cry, threw an armful of the little coats through the window. I looked in the mirror before I turned the corner of the drive; everybody was in tears.

Out on the road, I glanced down at the pathetic little animal gasping on the seat by my side. I patted the head and Tricki made a brave effort to wag his tail. "Poor old lad," I said, "you haven't a kick in you but I think I know a cure for you."

At the surgery, the household dogs surged round me. Tricki looked down at the noisy pack with dull eyes and, when put down, crouched motionless on the carpet. The other dogs, after sniffing round him for a few seconds, decided he was an uninteresting object and ignored him.

I made up a bed for him in a

warm loose box next to the one where the other dogs slept. For two days I kept an eye on him, giving him no food but plenty of water. At the end of the second day he started to show some interest in his surroundings and on the third he began to whimper when he heard the dogs in the yard.

When I opened the door, Tricki trotted out and was immediately engulfed by Joe the greyhound and his friends. After rolling him over and thoroughly inspecting him, the dogs moved off down the garden. Tricki followed them, rolling slightly with his surplus fat but obviously intrigued.

Later that day, I was present at feeding time. I watched while

Tristan slopped the food into the bowls. There was the usual headlong rush followed by the sounds of high-speed eating; every dog knew that if he fell behind the others he was liable to have some competition for the last part of his meal.

When they had finished, Tricki — who had taken no part in this — took a walk round the shining bowls, licking casually inside one or two of them. Next day, an extra bowl was put out for him and I was pleased to see him jostling his way toward it.

From then on, his progress was rapid. He had no medicinal treatment of any kind but all day he ran about with the dogs, joining in their friendly scrimmages. He discovered the joys of being bowled over, trampled on, and squashed every few minutes. He became an accepted member of the gang, an unlikely, silky little object among the shaggy crew, fighting like a tiger for his share at mealtimes and hunting rats in the old hen house at night. He had never had such a time in his life.

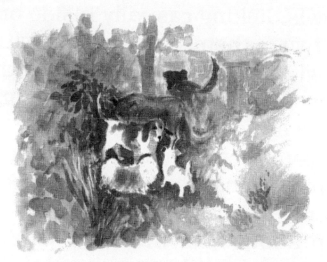

All the while, Mrs. Pumphrey hovered anxiously in the background, ringing a dozen times a day for the latest bulletins. I dodged the questions about whether his cushions were being turned regularly or his correct coat worn according to the weather; but I was able to tell her that the little fellow was out of danger and convalescing rapidly.

The word "convalescing" seemed to do something to Mrs. Pumphrey. She started to bring round fresh eggs, two dozen at a time to build up Tricki's strength. For a happy period there were two eggs each for breakfast, but when the bottles of sherry began to arrive, the real possibilities of the situation began to dawn on the household.

It was the same delicious brand that I knew so well and it was sent to enrich Tricki's blood. Lunch became a ceremonial occasion with two glasses before and several during the meal. Siegfried and Tristan took turns at proposing Tricki's health and the standard of speech-making improved daily. As the sponsor, I was always called upon to reply.

We could hardly believe it when the brandy came. Two bottles of Cordon Bleu, intended to put a final edge on Tricki's constitution. Siegfried dug out some balloon glasses belonging to his mother. I had never seen them before, but for a few nights they saw constant service as the fine spirit was rolled around, inhaled and reverently drunk.

They were days of deep content, starting well with the extra eggs in the morning, bolstered up and sustained by the midday sherry and finishing luxuriously round the fire with the brandy.

It was a temptation to keep Tricki on as a permanent guest, but I knew Mrs. Pumphrey was suffering and, after a fortnight, felt compelled to phone and tell her that the little dog had recovered and was awaiting collection.

Within minutes, about thirty feet of gleaming black metal drew up outside the surgery. The chauffeur opened the door and I could just make out the figure of

Mrs. Pumphrey almost lost in the interior. Her hands were tightly clasped in front of her; her lips trembled. "Oh, Mr. Herriot, do tell me the truth. Is he really better?"

"Yes, he's fine. There's no need for you to get out of the car — I'll go and fetch him."

I walked through the house into the garden. A mass of dogs was hurtling round and round the lawn and in their midst, ears flapping, tail waving, was the little golden figure of Tricki. In two weeks he had been transformed into a lithe, hard-muscled animal; he was keeping up well with the pack, stretching out in great bounds, his chest almost brushing the ground.

I carried him back along the

passage to the front of the house. The chauffeur was still holding the car door open and when Tricki saw his mistress he took off from my arms in a tremendous leap and sailed into Mrs. Pumphrey's lap. She gave a startled "Ooh!" and then had to defend herself as he swarmed over her, licking her face and barking.

During the excitement, I helped the chauffeur to bring out the beds, toys, cushions, coats, and bowls, none of which had been used. As the car moved away, Mrs. Pumphrey leaned out of the window. Tears shone in her eyes. Her lips trembled.

"Oh, Mr. Herriot," she cried, "how can I ever thank you? This is a triumph of surgery!"

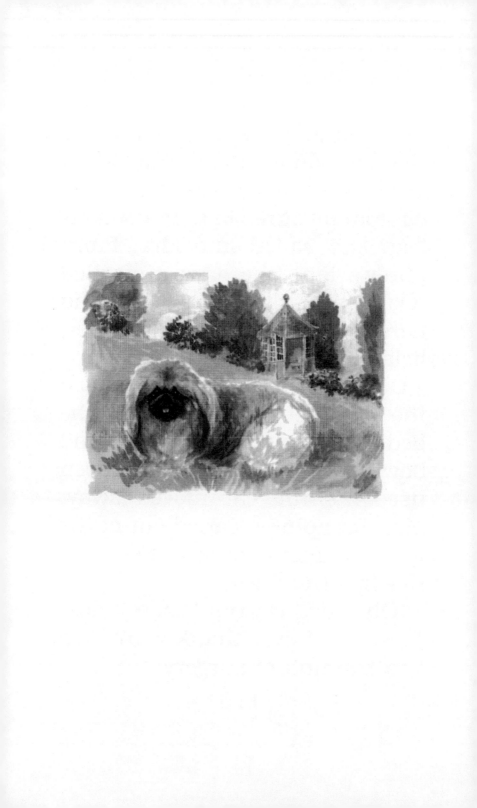

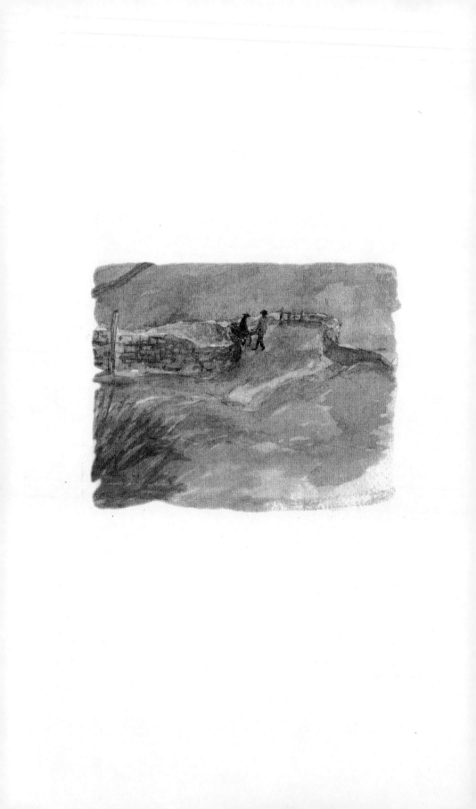

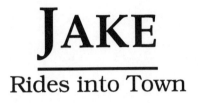

JAKE

Rides into Town

I suppose it isn't unusual to see a man pushing a pram in a town, but on a lonely moorland road the sight merits a second glance. Especially when the pram contains a large gray dog.

That was what I saw in the hills above Darrowby one morning and I slowed down as I drove past. I had noticed the strange combination before — on several occasions over the last few weeks — and it was clear that man and dog had recently moved into the district.

119

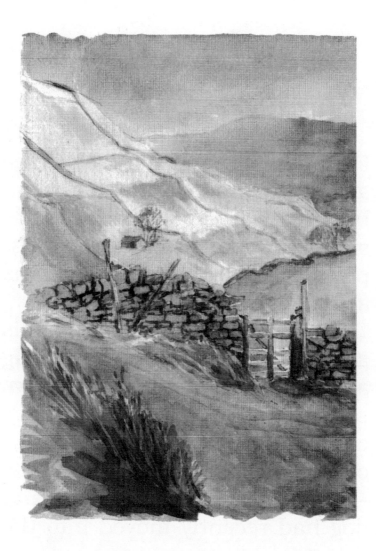

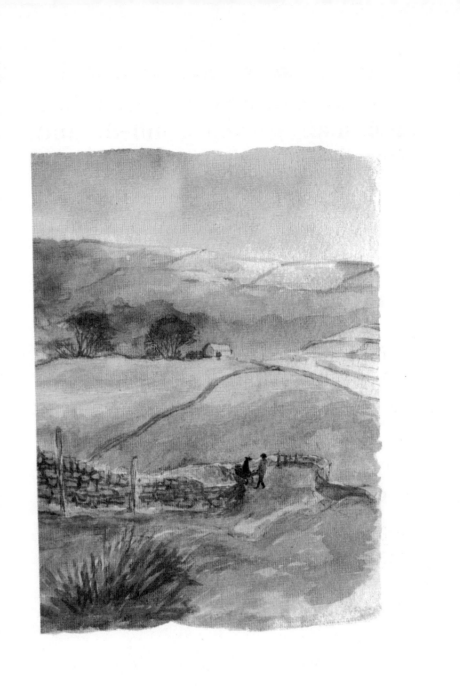

As the car drew abreast of him the man turned, smiled, and raised his hand. It was a smile of rare sweetness in a very brown face. A forty-year-old face, I thought, above a brown neck which bore neither collar nor tie, and a faded striped shirt lying open over a bare chest despite the coldness of the day.

I couldn't help wondering who or what he was. The outfit of scuffed suede golf jacket, corduroy trousers, and sturdy boots didn't give much clue. Some people might have put him down as an ordinary tramp, but there was a businesslike energetic look about him which didn't fit the term.

I wound the window down and

the thin wind of a Yorkshire March bit at my cheeks.

"Nippy this morning," I said.

The man seemed surprised. "Aye," he replied after a moment. "Aye, reckon it is."

I looked at the pram, ancient and rusty, and at the big animal sitting upright inside it. He was a lurcher, a cross-bred grey-hound, and he gazed back at me with unruffled dignity.

"Nice dog," I said.

"Aye, that's Jake." The man smiled again, showing good regular teeth. "He's a grand'un."

I waved and drove on. In the mirror I could see the compact figure stepping out briskly, head up, shoulders squared, and, rising like a statue from the middle of the pram, the huge brindled form of Jake.

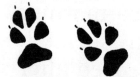

I didn't have to wait long to meet the unlikely pair again. I was examining a carthorse's teeth in a farmyard when on the hillside beyond the stable I saw a figure kneeling by a dry stone wall. And by his side, a pram and a big dog sitting patiently on the grass.

"Hey, just a minute," I pointed at the hill, "who is that?"

The farmer laughed. "That's Roddy Travers. D'you ken 'im?"

"No, no I don't. I had a word with him on the road the other day, that's all."

"Aye, on the road." He nodded

knowingly. "That's where you'd see Roddy, right enough."

"But what is he? Where does he come from?"

"He comes from somewhere in Yorkshire, but ah don't rightly know where and ah don't think anybody else does. But I'll tell you this — he can turn 'is hand to anything."

"Yes," I said, watching the man expertly laying the flat slabs of stone as he repaired a gap in the wall. "There's not many can do what he's doing now."

"That's true. Wallin' is a skilled job and it's dying out, but Roddy's a dab hand at it. But he can do owt — hedgin', ditchin', lookin' after stock, it's all the same to him."

I lifted the tooth rasp and began to rub a few sharp corners off the horse's molars. "And how long will he stay here?"

"Oh, when he's finished that wall he'll be off. Ah could do with 'im stoppin' around for a bit but he never stays in one place for long."

"But hasn't he got a home anywhere?"

"Nay, nay." The farmer laughed again. "Roddy's got nowt. All 'e has in the world is in that there pram."

Over the next weeks, as the harsh spring began to soften and the sunshine brought a bright speckle of primroses onto the grassy banks, I saw Roddy quite often, sometimes on the road, occasionally wielding a spade busily on the ditches around the fields. Jake was always there, either loping by his side or watching him at work. But we didn't actually meet again until I was inoculating Mr. Pawson's sheep.

There were three hundred to do and they were driven in batches into a small pen where Roddy caught and held them for me. And I could see he was an expert at this, too. The wild hill sheep whipped past him like bullets but he seized their fleece effortlessly, sometimes in midair, and held the foreleg up to expose that bare clean area of skin behind the elbow that nature seemed to provide for the veterinary surgeon's needle.

Outside on the windy slopes the

big lurcher sat upright in typical pose, looking with mild interest at the farm dogs prowling intently around the pens, but not interfering in any way.

"You've got him well trained," I said.

Roddy smiled. "Yes, ye'll never find Jake dashin' about, annoyin' people. He knows 'e has to sit there till I'm finished and there he'll sit."

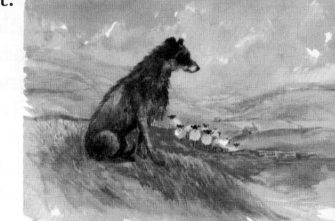

"And quite happy to do so, by

the look of him." I glanced again at the dog, a picture of content-ment. "He must live a wonderful life, traveling everywhere with you."

"You're right there," Mr. Pawson broke in as he ushered another bunch of sheep into the pen. "He hasn't a care in t'world, just like his master."

Roddy didn't say anything, but as the sheep ran in he straight-ened up and took a long steady breath. He had been working hard and a little trickle of sweat ran down the side of his forehead, but as he gazed over the wide sweep of moor and fell I could read utter serenity in his face. After a few moments he spoke.

"I reckon that's true. We haven't

much to worry us, Jake and me."

Mr. Pawson grinned mischievously. "By gaw, Roddy, you never spoke a truer word. No wife, no kids, no life insurance, no overdraft at t'bank — you must have a right peaceful existence."

"Ah suppose so," Roddy said. "But then ah've no money either."

The farmer gave him a quizzical look. "Aye, how about that, then? Wouldn't you feel a bit more secure, like, if you had a bit o' brass put by?"

"Nay, nay. Ye can't take it with you and, any road, as long as a man can pay 'is way, he's got enough."

There was nothing original about the words, but they have stayed with me all my life because they came from his lips and were spoken with such profound assurance.

When I had finished the inoculations and the ewes were turned out to trot back happily over the open fields I turned to Roddy. "Well, thanks very much. It makes my job a lot quicker when I have a good catcher like you." I pulled out a packet of Gold Flake. "Will you have a cigarette?"

"No, thank ye, Mr. Herriot. I don't smoke."

"You don't?"

"No — I don't drink either." He gave me his gentle smile and again I had the impression of physical and mental purity. No drinking, no smoking, a life of constant movement in the open air without material possessions or ambitions — it all showed in the unclouded eyes, the fresh skin and the hard, muscular frame. He wasn't very big but he looked indestructible.

"C'mon, Jake, it's dinnertime," he said and the big lurcher bounded around him in delight. I went over and spoke to the dog and he responded with tremendous body-swaying wags, his handsome face looking up at me, full of friendliness.

I stroked the long pointed head and tickled the ears. "He's a beauty, Roddy — a grand'un, as you said."

I walked to the house to wash my hands and before I went inside I glanced back at the two of them. They were sitting in the shelter of a wall and Roddy was laying out a thermos flask and a parcel of food while Jake watched eagerly. The hard bright sunshine beat on them as the wind whistled over the top of the wall. They looked supremely comfortable and at peace.

"He's independent, you see," the farmer's wife said as I stood at the kitchen sink. "He's welcome to come in for a bit o'dinner but he'd rather stay outside with his dog."

I nodded. "Where does he sleep when he's going round the farms like this?"

"Oh, anywhere," she replied. "In hay barns or granaries or sometimes out in the open, but when he's with us he sleeps upstairs in one of our rooms. Ah know for a fact any of the farmers would be willin' to have him in the house because he allus keeps himself spotless clean."

"I see." I pulled the towel from behind the door. "He's quite a character, isn't he?"

She smiled ruminatively. "Aye, he certainly is. Just him and his dog!" She lifted a fragrant dishful of hot roast ham from the oven and set it on the table. "But I'll tell you this. The feller's all right. Everybody likes Roddy Travers — he's a very nice man."

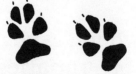

Roddy stayed around the Darrowby district throughout the summer and I grew used to the sight of him on the farms or pushing his pram along the roads. When it was raining he wore a tattered overlong gabardine coat, but at other times it was always the golf jacket and corduroys. I don't know where he had accumulated his wardrobe — but it was a safe bet that he had never been on a golf course in his life.

I saw him one morning on a hill path in early October. It had been a night of iron frost and the tussocky pastures beyond the walls were held in a pitiless white grip with every blade of grass stiffly ensheathed in rime.

I was muffled to the eyes and

had been beating my gloved fingers against my knees to thaw
them out, but when I pulled up
and wound down the window the
first thing I saw was the bare
chest under the collarless unbut-
toned shirt.

"Mornin', Mr. Herriot," he said.
"Ah'm glad I've seen ye." He
paused and gave me his tranquil
smile. "There's a job along t'road
for a couple of weeks, then I'm
movin' on."

"I see." I knew enough about
him now not to ask where he was
going. Instead I looked down at
Jake, who was sniffing the herb-
age. "I see he's walking this
morning."

Roddy laughed. "Yes, sometimes
'e likes to walk, sometimes 'e likes

136

to ride. He pleases 'imself."

"Right, Roddy," I said. "No doubt we'll meet again. All the best to you."

He waved and set off jauntily over the icebound road, and I felt that a little vein of richness had gone from my life.

But I was wrong. That same evening about eight o'clock the front doorbell rang. I answered it and found Roddy on the front door steps. Behind him, just visible in the frosty darkness, stood the ubiquitous pram.

"I want you to look at me dog, Mr. Herriot," he said.

"Why, what's the trouble?"

"Ah don't rightly know. He's havin' sort of . . . faintin' fits."

"Fainting fits? That doesn't

sound like Jake. Where is he, anyway?"

He pointed behind him. "In t'pram, under t'cover."

"All right." I threw the door wide. "Bring him in."

Roddy adroitly manhandled the rusty old vehicle up the steps and pushed it, squeaking and rattling, along the passage to the consulting room. There, under the bright lights, he snapped back the fasteners and threw off the cover to reveal Jake stretched beneath.

His head was pillowed on the familiar gabardine coat and around him lay his master's worldly goods: a string-tied bundle of spare shirt and socks, a packet of tea, a thermos, knife and spoon, and an ex-army haver-sack.

The big dog looked up at me with terrified eyes and as I patted him I could feel his whole frame quivering.

"Let him lie there a minute, Roddy," I said, "and tell me exactly what you've seen."

He rubbed his palms together and his fingers trembled. "Well, it only started this afternoon. He was right as rain, larkin' about on the grass, then he went into a sort o' fit."

"How do you mean?"

"Just kind of seized up and toppled over on 'is side. He lay there for a bit, gaspin' and slaverin'. Ah'll tell ye, I thought he was a goner." His eyes widened and a corner of his mouth twitched at the memory.

"How long did that last?"

"Nobbut a few seconds. Then he got up and you'd say there was nowt wrong with 'im."

"But he did it again?"

"Aye, time and time again. Drove me near daft. But in between 'e was normal. Normal, Mr. Herriot!"

It sounded ominously like the onset of epilepsy. "How old is he?" I asked.

"Five gone last February."

Ah well, it was a bit old for that. I reached for a stethoscope and listened intently to the heart but heard only the racing beat of a frightened animal. There was no abnormality. My thermometer showed no rise in temperature.

"Let's have him on the table, Roddy. You take the back end."

The big animal was limp in our arms as we hoisted him onto the smooth surface, but after lying there for a moment he looked timidly around him, then sat up with a slow and careful movement. As we watched he reached out and licked his master's face while his tail flickered between his legs.

"Look at that!" the man exclaimed. "He's all right again. You'd think he didn't ail a thing."

And indeed Jake was recovering his confidence rapidly. He peered tentatively at the floor a few times, then suddenly jumped down, trotted to his master, and put his paws against his chest.

I looked at the dog standing there, tail wagging furiously. "Well, that's a relief, anyway. I didn't like the look of him just then, but whatever's been troubling him seems to have righted itself. I'll . . ."

My happy flow was cut off. I started for the lurcher. His forelegs were on the floor again and his mouth was gaping as he fought for breath. Frantically he gasped and retched, then he blundered across the floor, collided with the pram wheels, and fell on his side.

"What the hell . . . ! Quick, get him up again!" I grabbed the animal round the middle and we lifted him back onto the table.

I watched in disbelief as the huge form lay there. There was no fight for breath now — he wasn't breathing at all, he was unconscious. I pushed my fingers along the inside of his thigh and felt the pulse. It was still going, rapid and feeble, but yet he didn't breathe.

He could die any moment and I stood there helpless, all my scientific training useless. Finally my frustration burst from me and I struck the dog on the ribs with the flat of my hand.

"Jake!" I yelled, "Jake, what's the matter with you?"

As though in reply, the lurcher immediately started to take great wheezing breaths, his eyelids twitched back to consciousness, and he began to look about him. But he was still mortally afraid and he lay prone as I gently stroked his tousled head.

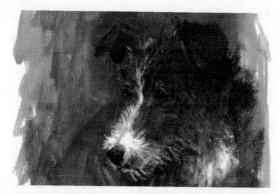

There was a long silence while the animal's terror slowly subsided, then he sat up on the table, looked round the room, and finally regarded us placidly.

"There you are," Roddy said softly. "Same thing again. Ah can't reckon it up and ah thought ah knew summat about dogs."

I didn't say anything. I couldn't

reckon it up either, and I was supposed to be a veterinary surgeon.

I spoke at last. "Roddy, that wasn't a fit. He was choking. Something was interfering with his air flow." I took my hand torch from my breast pocket. "I'm going to have a look at his throat."

I pushed Jake's jaws apart, depressed his tongue with a forefinger, and shown the light into the depths. He was the kind of good-natured dog who offered no resistance as I prodded around, but despite my floodlit view of the pharynx I could find nothing wrong. I had been hoping desperately to come across a bit of bone stuck there somewhere, but I ranged feverishly over pink

145

tongue, healthy tonsils, and gleaming molars without success. Everything looked perfect.

I was tilting his head a little farther when I felt him stiffen and heard Roddy's cry.

"He's goin' again!"

And he was, too. I stared in horror as the brindled body slid away from me and lay prostrate once more on the table. And again the mouth strained wide and froth bubbled round the lips. As before, the breathing had stopped and the rib cage was motionless. As the seconds ticked away I beat on the chest with my hand but it didn't work this time. I pulled the lower eyelid down from the staring orb — the conjunctiva was blue, Jake hadn't long to live. The tragedy of the thing bore down on me. This wasn't just a dog, he was this man's family and I was watching him die.

It was at that moment that I heard the faint sound. It was a strangled cough which barely stirred the dog's lips.

"Damn it!" I shouted. "He is choking. There must be something down there."

Again I seized the head and pushed my torch into the mouth, and I shall always be thankful that at that very instant the dog coughed again, opening up the cartilages of the larynx and giving me a glimpse of the cause of all the trouble. There, beyond the drooping epiglottis, I saw for a fleeting moment a smooth round object no bigger than a pea.

"I think it's a pebble," I gasped. "Right inside his larynx."

"You mean, in 'is Adam's apple?"

"That's right, and it's acting like a ball valve, blocking his windpipe every now and then." I shook the dog's head. "You see, look, I've dislodged it for the moment. He's coming round again."

Once more Jake was reviving and breathing steadily.

Roddy ran his hand over the head, along the back and down the great muscles of the hind limbs. "But . . . but . . . it'll happen again, won't it?"

I nodded. "I'm afraid so."

"And one of these times it isn't

goin' to shift and that'll be the end of 'im?" He had gone very pale.

"That's about it, Roddy. I'll have to get that pebble out."

"But how . . . ?"

"Cut into the larynx. And right now — it's the only way."

"All right," he swallowed. "Let's get on. I don't think ah could stand it if he went down again."

I knew what he meant. My knees had begun to shake, and I had a strong conviction that if Jake collapsed once more then so would I.

I seized a pair of scissors and clipped away the hair from the ventral surface of the larynx. I dared not use a general anesthetic, and therefore I infiltrated

the area with local before swab-
bing with antiseptic. Mercifully
there was a freshly boiled set of
instruments lying in the steril-
izer, and I lifted out the tray and
set it on the trolley by the side of
the table.

"Hold his head steady," I said
hoarsely, and gripped a scalpel.

I cut down through skin, fascia,
and the thin layers of the muscle
until the ventral surface of the
larynx was revealed. This was
something I had never done to a
live dog before, but desperation
abolished any hesitancy and it
took me only another few seconds
to incise the thin membrane and
peer into the interior.

And there it was. A pebble right
enough — gray and glistening

and tiny, but big enough to kill.

I had to fish it out quickly and cleanly without pushing it into the trachea. I leaned back and rummaged in the tray until I found some broad-bladed forceps, then I poised them over the wound. Great surgeons' hands, I felt sure, didn't shake like this, nor did such men pant as I was doing. But I clenched my teeth, introduced the forceps, and my hand magically steadied as I clamped them over the pebble.

I stopped panting, too. In fact I didn't breathe at all as I bore the shining little object slowly and tenderly through the opening and dropped it with a gentle rat-tat on the table.

"Is that it?" asked Roddy, almost in a whisper.

"That's it." I reached for needle and suture silk. "All is well now."

The stitching took only a few minutes and by the end of it Jake was bright-eyed and alert, paws shifting impatiently, ready for anything. He seemed to know his troubles were over.

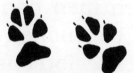

Roddy brought him back in ten days to have the stitches re-moved. It was, in fact, the very morning he was leaving the Dar-rowby district, and after I had picked the few loops of silk from the nicely healed wound I walked with him to the front door while Jake capered round our feet.

On the pavement outside Skeldale House the ancient pram stood in all its high, rusted dignity. Roddy pulled back the cover.

"Up, boy," he murmured, and the big dog leaped effortlessly into his accustomed place.

Roddy took hold of the handle with both hands and as the autumn sunshine broke suddenly through the clouds it lit up a picture which had grown familiar and part of the daily scene. The golf jacket, the open shirt and brown chest, the handsome animal sitting up, looking around him with natural grace.

"Well, so long, Roddy," I said. "I suppose you'll be round these parts again."

He turned and I saw that smile

again. "Aye, reckon ah'll be back."

He gave a push and they were off, the strange vehicle creaking, Jake swaying gently as they went down the street. The memory came back to me of what I had seen under the cover that night in the surgery. The haversack, which would contain his razor, towel, soap, and a few other things. The packet of tea and the thermos. And something else — a tiny dog collar. Could it have belonged to Jake as a pup or to another loved animal? It added a little more mystery to the man . . . and explained other things, too. That farmer had been right — all Roddy possessed was in that pram.

And it seemed it was all he

desired, too, because as he turned the corner and disappeared from my view I could hear him whistling.

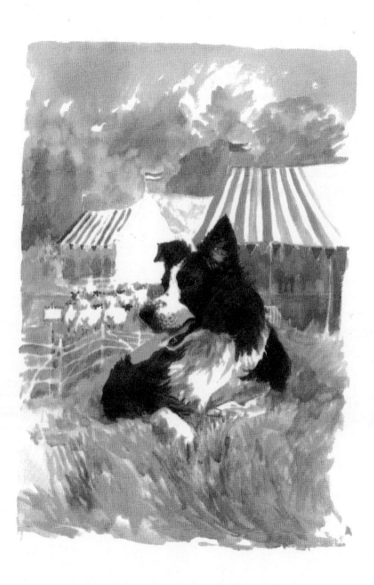

GYP

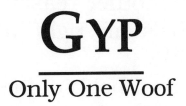

Only One Woof

"Is this what you've been telling me about, Mr. Wilkin?" I asked the farmer who was gazing down at his dog.

The farmer nodded, "Aye, that's it, it's always like that, always the same."

I looked down at the helpless convulsions of the big dog lying at my feet; at the staring eyes, the wildly pedaling limbs. The farmer had told me about the periodic attacks which had begun to affect his sheepdog, Gyp, but it was coincidence that one should occur when I was on the farm for another reason.

"And he's all right afterward, you say?"

"Right as a bobbin. Seems a bit dazed, maybe, for about an hour, then he's back to normal." The farmer shrugged. "I've had lots o' dogs through my hands, as you know, and I've seen plenty of dogs with fits. I thought I knew all the causes — worms, wrong feeding, distemper — but this has me beat. I've tried everything."

"Well, you can stop trying, Mr. Wilkin," I said. "You won't be able to do much for Gyp. He's got epilepsy."

"Epilepsy? But he's a grand, normal dog most of t'time."

"Yes, I know. That's how it goes.

158

There's nothing actually wrong with his brain — it's a mysterious condition. The cause is unknown but it's almost certainly hereditary."

Mr. Wilkin raised his eyebrows. "Well that's a rum 'un. If it's hereditary why hasn't it shown up before now? He's nearly two years old and he didn't start this till a few months ago."

"That's typical," I replied. "Eighteen months to two years is about the time it usually appears."

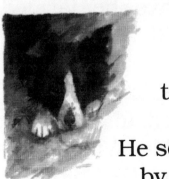

Gyp interrupted us by getting up and staggering toward his master, wagging his tail. He seemed untroubled by his experience. In fact the whole thing had lasted less than two minutes.

Mr. Wilkin bent and stroked the rough head briefly. His craggy features were set in a thoughtful cast. He was a big, powerful man in his forties, and now, as the eyes narrowed in that face which rarely smiled, he looked almost menacing. I had heard more than one man say he wouldn't like to get on the wrong side of Sep Wilkin, and I could see what they meant. But he had always treated me right and since he farmed nearly a thousand acres I saw quite a lot of him.

His passion was sheepdogs. A lot of farmers liked to run dogs at the trials but Mr. Wilkin was one of the top men. He bred and trained dogs which regularly won at the local events and occasionally at the national trials. And what was troubling me was that Gyp was his main hope.

He had picked out the two best pups from a litter — Gyp and Sweep — and had trained them with the dedication that had made him a winner. I don't think I have ever seen two dogs enjoy each other quite as much; whenever I was on the farm I would see them together, sometimes peeping nose by nose over the half door of the loose box where they slept, occasionally slinking devotedly round the feet of their master but usually just playing together. They must have spent hours rolling about in ecstatic wrestling matches, growling and panting, gnawing gently at each other's limbs.

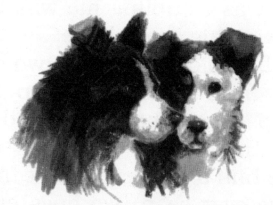

A few months ago George Crossley, one of Mr. Wilkin's oldest friends and a keen trial man, had lost his best dog with nephritis and Mr. Wilkin had let him have Sweep. I was surprised at the time because Sweep was shaping better than Gyp in his training and looked as if he would turn out a real champion. But it was Gyp who remained. He must have missed his friend but there were other dogs on the farm, and if they didn't quite make up for Sweep he was never really lonely.

As I watched, I could see the dog recovering rapidly. It was extraordinary how soon normality was restored after that frightening convulsion. And I waited with some apprehension to hear what his master would say.

The cold, logical decision for him to make would be to have Gyp put down and, looking at the friendly, tail-wagging animal, I didn't like the idea at all. There was something very attractive about him. The big-boned, well-marked body was handsome, but his most distinctive feature was his head where one ear somehow contrived to stick up while the other lay flat, giving him a lop-sided, comic appeal. Gyp, in fact, looked a bit of a clown. But a clown who radiated goodwill and camaraderie.

Mr. Wilkin spoke at last. "Will he get any better as he grows older?"

"Almost certainly not," I replied.

"Then he'll always 'ave these fits?"

"I'm afraid so. You say he has them every two or three weeks — well, it will probably carry on more or less like that with occasional variations."

"But he could have one any time?"

"Yes."

"In the middle of a trial, like." The farmer sunk his head on his chest and his voice rumbled deep. "That's it, then."

In the long silence which followed, the fateful words became more and more inevitable. Sep Wilkin wasn't the man to hesitate in a matter which concerned his ruling passion. Ruthless culling of any animal which didn't come up to standard would be his policy. When he finally cleared his throat I had a sinking premonition of what he was going to say.

But I was wrong.

"If I kept him, could you do anything for him?" he asked.

"Well, I could give you some pills for him. They might decrease the frequency of the fits." I tried to keep the eagerness out of my voice.

"Right . . . right . . . I'll come into t'surgery and get some," he muttered.

"Fine. But . . . er . . . you won't ever breed from him, will you?" I said.

"Naw, naw, naw," the farmer grunted with a touch of irritability as though he didn't want to pursue the matter further.

And I held my peace because I felt intuitively that he did not want to be detected in a weakness; that he was prepared to keep the dog simply as a pet. It was funny how events began to slot into place and suddenly make sense. That was why he had let Sweep, the superior trial dog, go. He just liked Gyp. In fact Sep Wilkin, hard man though he may be, had succumbed to that offbeat charm.

So I shifted to some light chatter about the weather as I walked back to the car, but when I was about to drive off the farmer returned to the main subject.

"There's one thing about Gyp I never mentioned," he said, bending to the window. "I don't know whether it has owt to do with the job or not. He has never barked in his life."

I looked at him in surprise. "You mean never, ever?"

"That's right. Not a single bark. T'other dogs make a noise when strangers come on the farm but I've never heard Gyp utter a sound since he was born."

"Well, that's very strange," I said. "But I can't see that it is connected with his condition in any way."

As I switched on the engine I noticed for the first time that while a bitch and two half-grown pups gave tongue to see me on my way Gyp merely regarded me in his comradely way.

The thing intrigued me. So much so that whenever I was on the farm over the next few months I made a point of watching the big sheepdog at whatever he was doing. But there was never any change. Between the convulsions which had settled down to around three-week intervals he was a normal, active, happy animal. But soundless.

I saw him, too, in Darrowby when his master came in to market. Gyp was often seated comfortably in the back of the car, but if I happened to speak to Mr. Wilkin on these occasions I kept off the subject because, as I said, I had the feeling that he more than most farmers would hate to be exposed in keeping a dog for other than working purposes.

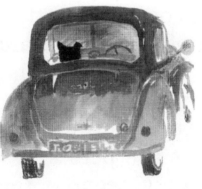

And yet I have always entertained a suspicion that most farm dogs were more or less pets. The dogs on sheep farms were of course indispensable working animals and on other establishments they no doubt performed a function in helping to bring in the cows. But watching them on my daily rounds I often wondered. I saw them rocking along on carts at haytime, chasing rats among the stooks at harvest, pottering around the buildings or roaming the fields at the side of the farmer; and I wondered . . . what did they really do?

I still stick to my theory: most farm dogs are pets and they are there mainly because the farmer just likes to have them around.

You would have to put a farmer on the rack to get him to admit it but I think I am right. And in the process those dogs have a wonderful time. They don't have to beg for walks, they are out all day long, and in the company of their masters. If I want to find a man on a farm I look for his dog, knowing the man won't be far away. I try to give my own dogs a good life but it cannot compare with the life of the average farm dog.

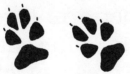

There was a long spell when Sep Wilkin's stock stayed healthy and I didn't see either him or Gyp, then I came across them both by accident at a sheepdog trial. It was a local event, run in conjunction with the Mellerton Agricultural Show, and since I was in the district I decided to steal an hour off.

I took Helen with me, too, because these trials have always fascinated us. The wonderful control of the owners over their animals, the intense involvement of the dogs themselves, the sheer skill of the whole operation always held us spellbound.

She put her arm through mine as we went in at the entrance gate to where a crescent of cars was drawn up at one end of a long field. The field was on the river's edge and through a fringe of trees the afternoon sunshine glinted on the tumbling water of the shallows and turned the long beach of bleached stones to a dazzling white. Groups of men, mainly competitors, stood around chatting as they watched. They were quiet, easy, bronzed men, and as they seemed to be drawn from all social strata from prosperous farmers to working men their garb was varied: cloth caps, trilbies, deerstalkers, or no hat at all; tweed jackets, stiff best suits, open-necked shirts, fancy ties, sometimes neither collar nor tie. Nearly all of them leaned on long crooks with the handles fashioned from rams' horns.

Snatches of talk reached us as we walked among them.

"You got 'ere, then, Fred."

"That's a good gather." "Nay, 'e's missed one, 'e'll get nowt for that." "Them sheep's a bit flighty." "Aye, they're buggers." And above it all the whistles of the man running a dog; every conceivable level and pitch of whistle with now and then a shout. "Sit!" "Get by!" Every man had his own way with his dog.

The dogs waiting their turn were tied up to a fence with a hedge growing over it. There were about seventy of them and it was rather wonderful to see that long row of waving tails and friendly expressions. They were mostly strangers to each other but there wasn't even the semblance of disagreement, never mind a fight. It seemed that the natural obedience of these little creatures was linked to an amicable disposition.

This appeared to be common to their owners, too. There was no animosity, no resentment at defeat, no unseemly display of triumph in victory. If a man overran his time he ushered his group of sheep quietly in the corner and returned with a philosophical grin to his colleagues. There was a little quiet leg-pulling but that was all.

We came across Sep Wilkin leaning against his car at the best vantage point about thirty yards away from the final pen. Gyp, tied to the bumper, turned and gave me his crooked grin while Mrs. Wilkin on a camp stool by his side rested a hand on his shoulder. Gyp, it seemed, had got under her skin too.

Helen went over to speak to her and I turned to her husband. "Are you running a dog today, Mr. Wilkin?"

"No, not this time, just come to watch, but I know a lot o' the dogs."

I stood near him for a while watching the action, breathing in the clean smell of trampled grass and plug tobacco. In front of us next to the pen the judge stood by his post.

I had been there for about ten minutes when Mr. Wilkin lifted a pointed finger. "Look who's there!"

George Crossley with Sweep

trotting at his heels was making his way unhurriedly to the post. Gyp suddenly stiffened and sat up very straight, his cocked ears accentuating the lopsided look. It was many months since he had seen his brother and companion; it seemed unlikely, I thought, that he would remember him. But his interest was clearly intense, and as the judge waved his white handkerchief and the three sheep were released from the far corner he rose slowly to his feet.

A gesture from Mr. Crossley sent Sweep winging round the perimeter of the field in a wide, joyous gallop, and as he neared the sheep a whistle dropped him on his belly. From then on it was an object lesson in the cooperation of man and dog. Sep Wilkin had always said Sweep would be a champion and he looked the part, darting and falling at his master's commands. Short piercing whistles, shrill plaintive whistles; he was in tune with them all.

No dog all day had brought his sheep through the three lots of gates as effortlessly as Sweep did now, and as he approached the pen near us it was obvious that he would win the cup unless some disaster struck. But this was the touchy bit; more than once with other dogs the sheep had broken free and gone bounding away within feet of the wooden rails.

George Crossley held the gate

178

wide and extended his crook. You could see now why they all carried those long sticks. His commands to Sweep, huddled flat along the turf, were now almost inaudible, but the quiet words brought the dog inching first one way, then the other. The sheep were in the entrance to the pen now but they still looked around them irresolutely and the game was not over yet. But as Sweep wriggled toward them almost imperceptibly they turned and entered and Mr. Crossley crashed the gate behind them.

As he did so he turned to Sweep with a happy cry of *"Good lad!"* and the dog responded with a quick jerking wag of his tail.

At that, Gyp, who had been

standing very tall, watching every move with the most intense concentration, raised his head and emitted a single resounding bark.

"*Woof!*" went Gyp — and we all stared at him in astonishment.

"Did you hear that?" gasped Mrs. Wilkin.

"Well, by gaw!" her husband burst out, looking openmouthed at his dog.

Gyp didn't seem to be aware that he had done anything unusual. He was too preoccupied by the reunion with his brother and within seconds the two dogs were rolling around, chewing playfully at each other as of old.

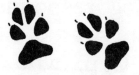

I suppose the Wilkins as well as myself had the feeling that this event might start Gyp barking like any other dog, but it was not to be.

Six years later I was on the farm and went to the house to get some hot water. As Mrs. Wilkin handed me the bucket she looked down at Gyp, who was basking in the sunshine outside the kitchen window.

"There you are, then, funny fellow," she said to the dog.

I laughed. "Has he ever barked since that day?"

Mrs. Wilkin shook her head. "No, he hasn't, not a sound. I waited a long time but I know he's not going to do it now."

"Ah well, it's not important. But

still, I'll never forget that afternoon at the trial," I said.

"Nor will I!" She looked at Gyp
again and her eyes softened in
reminiscence. "Poor old lad, eight
years old and only one woof!"

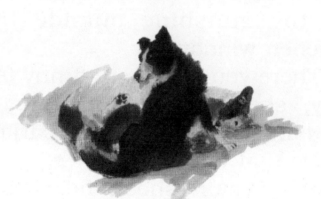

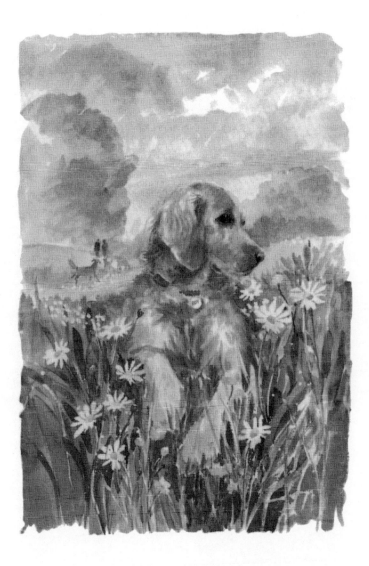

ROY

From Rags to Riches

The silver-haired old gentleman with the pleasant face didn't look the type to be easily upset, but his eyes glared at me angrily and his lips quivered with indignation.

"Mr. Herriot," he said, "I have come to make a complaint. I strongly object to your allowing my dog to suffer unnecessarily."

"Suffer? What suffering?"

"I think you know, Mr. Herriot. I brought my dog in a few days ago. He was very lame and I am referring to your treatment on that occasion."

185

I nodded. "Yes, I remember it well . . . but where does the suffering come in?"

"Well, the poor animal is going around with his leg dangling and I have it on good authority that the bone is fractured and should have been put in plaster immediately." The old gentleman stuck his chin out fiercely.

"All right, you can stop worrying," I said. "Your dog has a radial paralysis caused by a blow on the ribs and if you are patient and follow my treatment he'll gradually improve. In fact, I think he'll recover completely."

"But he trails his leg when he walks."

"I know — that's typical, and to the layman it does give the appearance of a broken leg. But he shows no sign of pain?"

"No, he seems quite happy, but this lady seemed to be absolutely sure of her facts. She was adamant."

"Lady?"

"Yes," said the old gentleman. "She is very clever with animals and she came round to see if she could help in my dog's convalescence. She brought some excellent condition powders with her."

"Ah!" A blinding shaft pierced the fog in my mind. All was suddenly clear. "It was Mrs. Donovan, wasn't it?"

"Well . . . er, yes. That was her name."

Old Mrs. Donovan was a woman who really got around. No

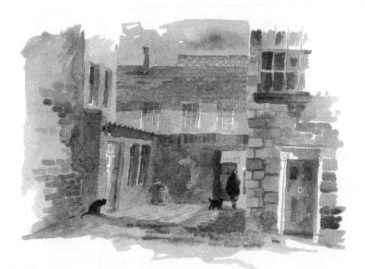

matter what was going on in Darrowby — weddings, funerals,
house sales — you'd find the
dumpy little figure and walnut
face among the spectators, the
darting, black-button eyes taking
everything in. And always, on the
end of its lead, her terrier dog.

When I say "old," I'm only
guessing, because she appeared
ageless; she seemed to have been
around a long time but she could

have been anything between fifty-five and seventy-five. She certainly had the vitality of a young woman because she must have walked vast distances in her dedicated quest to keep abreast of events. Many people took an uncharitable view of her acute curiosity, but whatever the motivation, her activities took her into almost every channel of life in the town. One of these channels was our veterinary practice.

Because Mrs. Donovan, among her other widely ranging interests, was an animal doctor. In fact I think it would be safe to say that this facet of her life

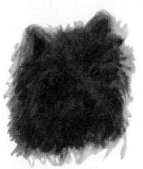

transcended all the others.

She could talk at length on the ailments of small animals and she had a whole armory of medicines and remedies at her command, her two specialties being her miracle-working condition powders and a dog shampoo of unprecedented value for improving the coat. She had an uncanny ability to sniff out a sick animal and it was not uncommon when I was on my rounds to find Mrs. Donovan's dark gypsy face poised intently over what I had thought was my patient while she administered calf's-foot jelly or one of her own patent nostrums.

I suffered more than Siegfried because I took a more active part in the small animal side of our practice. I was anxious to develop this aspect and to improve my image in this field and Mrs. Donovan didn't help at all. "Young Mr. Herriot," she would confide to my clients, "is all right with cattle and such like, but he don't know nothing about dogs and cats."

And of course they believed her and had implicit faith in her. She had the irresistible mystic appeal of the amateur and on top of that there was her habit, particularly endearing in Darrowby, of never charging for her advice, her medicines, or her long periods of diligent nursing.

Older folk in the town told how her husband, an Irish farm worker, had died many years ago and how he must have had a "bit put away" because Mrs. Donovan had apparently been able to indulge all her interests over the years without financial strain. Since she inhabited the streets of Darrowby all day and every day I often encountered her and she always smiled up at me sweetly and told me how she had been sitting up all night with Mrs. So-and-so's dog that I'd been treating. She felt sure she'd be able to pull it through.

There was no smile on her face, however, on the day when she rushed into the surgery while Siegfried and I were having tea.

"Mr. Herriot!" she gasped. "Can you come? My little dog's been run over!"

I jumped up and ran out to the car with her. She sat in the passenger seat with her head bowed, her hands clasped tightly on her knees.

"He slipped his collar and ran in front of a car," she murmured. "He's lying in front of the school halfway up Cliffend Road. Please hurry."

I was there within three minutes but as I bent over the dusty little body stretched out on the pavement I knew there was nothing I could do. The fast-glazing eyes, the faint, gasping respirations, the ghastly pallor of the mucous membranes all told the same story.

"I'll take him back to the surgery and get some saline into

him, Mrs. Donovan," I said, "but I'm afraid he's had a massive internal hemorrhage. Did you see what happened exactly?"

She gulped. "Yes, the wheel went right over him."

Ruptured liver, for sure. I passed my hands under the little animal and began to lift him gently, but as I did so the breathing stopped and the eyes stared fixedly ahead.

Mrs. Donovan sank to her knees and for a few moments she gently stroked the rough hair of the head and chest. "He's dead, isn't he?" she whispered at last.

"I'm afraid he is," I said.

She got slowly to her feet and stood bewilderedly among the little group of bystanders on the pavement. Her lips moved but she seemed unable to say anymore.

I took her arm, led her over to the car, and opened the door. "Get in and I'll run you home. Leave everything to me."

I wrapped the dog in an overall and laid him in the trunk before driving away. It wasn't until we drew up outside Mrs. Donovan's house that she began to weep silently. I sat there without speaking until she had finished. Then she wiped her eyes and turned to me.

"Do you think he suffered at all?"

"I'm certain he didn't. It was all so quick — he wouldn't have known a thing about it."

She tried to smile. "Poor little Rex. I don't know what I'm going to do without him. We've traveled a few miles together, you know."

"Yes, you have. He had a wonderful life, Mrs. Donovan. And let me give you a bit of advice — you must get another dog. You'd be lost without one."

She shook her head. "No, I couldn't. That little dog meant too much to me. I couldn't let another take his place."

"Well, I know that's how you feel just now, but I wish you'd think about it. I don't want to seem callous — I tell everybody this when they lose an animal and I know it's good advice."

"Mr. Herriot, I'll never have another one." She shook her head again, very decisively. "Rex was my faithful friend for many years and I just want to remember him. He's the last dog I'll ever have."

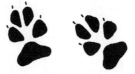

I often saw Mrs. Donovan around town after this and I was glad to see she was still as active as ever, though she looked strangely incomplete without the little dog on its lead. But it must have been over a month before I had the chance to speak to her.

It was on the afternoon that Inspector Halliday of the RSPCA rang me.

"Mr. Herriot," he said, "I'd like you to come and see an animal with me. A dog, and it's pretty

grim. A dreadful case of neglect."
He gave me the name of a row of
old brick cottages down by the
river and said he'd meet me there.

Halliday was waiting for me,
smart and businesslike in his
dark uniform, as I pulled up in
the back lane behind the houses.
He was a big blond man with
cheerful blue eyes, but he didn't
smile as he came over to the car.

"He's in here," he said, and led
the way toward one of the doors
in the long, crumbling wall. A few
curious people were hanging
around, and with a feeling of in-
evitability I recognized a gnome-
like brown face. Trust Mrs.
Donovan, I thought, to be among
those present at a time like this.

We went through the door into

the long garden. I had found that even the lowliest dwellings in Darrowby had long strips of land at the back as though the builders had taken it for granted that the country people who were going to live in them would want a bit of land for vegetable and fruit growing, even stock keeping in a small way. You usually found a pig there, a few hens, often pretty beds of flowers.

But this garden was a wilderness. A chilling air of desolation hung over the few gnarled apple and plum trees standing among a tangle of rank grass as though the place had been forsaken by all living creatures.

Halliday went over to a ramshackle wooden shed with peeling paint and a rusted corrugated iron roof. He produced a key, unlocked the padlock and dragged the door partly open. There was no window and it wasn't easy to identify the jumble inside; broken gardening tools, an ancient mangle, rows of flowerpots and partly used paint tins. And right at the back, a dog sitting quietly.

I didn't notice him immediately because of the gloom and because the smell in the shed started me coughing, but as I drew closer I saw that he was a big animal, sitting very upright, his collar secured by a chain to a ring in the wall. I had seen some thin dogs but this advanced emaciation reminded me of my textbooks on anatomy; nowhere else did the bones of pelvis, face, and rib cage stand out with such horrifying clarity. A deep, smoothed-out hollow in the earth floor showed where he had lain, moved about, in fact lived for a very long time.

The sight of the animal had a stupefying effect on me; I only half took in the rest of the scene — the filthy shreds of sacking scattered nearby, the bowl of scummy water.

There were sores all over his body, but his hindquarters were the worst. The coat, which seemed to be a dull yellow, was matted and caked with dirt.

The Inspector spoke again. "I don't think he's ever been out of here. He's only a young dog —

about a year old — but I understand he's been in this shed since he was an eight-week-old pup. Somebody out in the lane heard a cry or he'd never have been found."

I felt a tightening of the throat and a sudden nausea which wasn't due to the smell. It was the thought of this patient animal sitting starved and forgotten in the darkness and filth for a year. I looked again at the dog and saw in his eyes only a calm trust. Some dogs would have barked their heads off and soon been discovered, some would have become terrified and vicious, but this was one of the totally undemanding kind, the kind which had complete faith in people and accepted all their actions without complaint. Just an occasional whimper perhaps as he sat interminably in the empty blackness which had been his world and at times wondered what it was all about.

"Well, Inspector, I hope you're going to throw the book at whoever's responsible," I said.

Halliday grunted. "Oh, there won't be much done. It's a case of diminished responsibility. The owner's definitely simple, living with an aged mother. I've seen the fellow and it seems he threw in a bit of food when he felt like it and that's about all he did. They'll fine him and stop him keeping an animal in the future but nothing more than that."

"I see." I reached out and stroked the dog's head and he immediately responded by resting a paw on my wrist. There was a pathetic dignity about the way he held himself erect, the calm eyes regarding me, friendly and unafraid. "Well, you'll let me know if you want me in court."

"Of course, and thank you for coming along." Halliday hesitated for a moment. "And now I expect you'll want to put this poor thing out of his misery right away."

I continued to run my hand over the head and ears while I thought for a moment. "Yes . . . yes, I suppose so. We'd never find a home for him in this state. It's the kindest thing to do. Anyway, push the door wide open, will you, so that I can get a proper look at him."

In the improved light I examined him more thoroughly. Perfect teeth, well-proportioned limbs with a fringe of yellow hair. I put my stethoscope on his chest and as I listened to the slow, strong thudding of the heart the dog again put his paw on my hand.

I turned to Halliday. "You know, Inspector, inside this bag of bones there's a lovely healthy golden retriever. I wish there was some way of letting him out."

As I spoke I noticed there was more than one figure in the door opening. A pair of black pebble eyes was peering intently at the dog from behind the Inspector's broad back. The other spectators had remained in the lane but Mrs. Donovan's curiosity had been too much for her. I continued conversationally as though I hadn't seen her.

"You know, what this dog needs first of all is a good shampoo to clean up his matted coat."

"Huh?" said Halliday.

"Yes. And then he wants a long course of some really strong condition powders."

"What's that?" The Inspector looked startled.

"There's no doubt about it," I said. "It's the only hope for him, but where are you going to find such things? Really powerful enough, I mean." I sighed and straightened up. "Ah well, I suppose there's nothing else for it. I'd better put him to sleep right away. I'll get the things from my car."

When I got back to the shed Mrs. Donovan was already inside examining the dog despite the feeble remonstrances of the big man.

"Look!" she said excitedly, pointing to a name roughly scratched on the collar. "His name's Roy." She smiled up at me. "It's a bit like Rex, isn't it, that name."

"You know, Mrs. Donovan, now you mention it, it is. It's very like Rex, the way it comes off your tongue." I nodded seriously.

She stood silent for a few moments, obviously in the grip of a deep emotion, then she burst out.

207

"Can I have 'im? I can make him better, I know I can. Please, please let me have 'im!"

"Well, I don't know," I said. "It's really up to the Inspector. You'll have to get his permission."

Halliday looked at her in bewilderment, then he said: "Excuse me, madam," and drew me to one side. We walked a few yards through the long grass and stopped under a tree.

"Mr. Herriot," he whispered, "I don't know what's going on here, but I can't just pass over an animal in this condition to anybody who has a casual whim. The poor beggar's had one bad break already — I think it's enough. This woman doesn't look a suitable person . . ."

I held up my hand. "Believe me, Inspector, you've nothing to worry about. She's a funny old stick but she's been sent from heaven today. If anybody in Darrowby can give this dog a new life it's her."

Halliday still looked very doubtful. "But I still don't get it. What was all that stuff about him needing shampoos and condition powders?"

"Oh, never mind about that. I'll tell you some other time. What he needs is lots of good grub, care, and affection, and that's just what he'll get. You can take my word for it."

"All right, you seem very sure." Halliday looked at me for a second or two, then turned and walked over to the eager little figure by the shed.

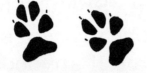

I had never before been deliberately on the lookout for Mrs. Donovan: she had just cropped up wherever I happened to be, but now I scanned the streets of Darrowby anxiously day by day without seeing her. I didn't like it when Gobber Newhouse got drunk and drove his bicycle determinedly through a barrier into a ten-foot hole where they were laying the new sewer and Mrs. Donovan was not in evidence among the happy crowd who watched the council workmen and two policemen trying to get him out; and when she was no-where to be seen when they had to fetch the fire engine to the fish and chip shop the night the fat burst into flames, I became seri-ously worried.

Maybe I should have called round to see how she was getting on with that dog. Certainly I had trimmed off the dead tissue and dressed the sores before she took him away, but perhaps he needed something more than that. And yet at the time I had felt a strong conviction that the main thing was to get him out of there and clean him and feed him and na-ture would do the rest. And I had a lot of faith in Mrs. Donovan — far more than she had in me — when it came to animal doctoring;

it was hard to believe I'd been completely wrong.

It must have been nearly three weeks and I was on the point of calling her at home when I noticed her stumping briskly along the far side of the marketplace, peering closely into every shop window exactly as before. The only difference was that she had a big yellow dog on the end of the lead.

I turned the wheel and sent my car bumping over the cobbles till I was abreast of her. When she saw me getting out she stopped and smiled impishly but she didn't speak as I bent over Roy and examined him. He was still a skinny dog but he looked bright and happy, his wounds were healing healthily, and there was not a speck of dirt in his coat or on his skin. I knew then what Mrs. Donovan had been doing all this time; she had been washing and combing and teasing at that filthy tangle until she finally conquered it.

As I straightened up she seized my wrist in a grip of surprising strength and looked up into my eyes.

"Now, Mr. Herriot," she said, "haven't I made a difference to this dog!"

"You've done wonders, Mrs. Donovan," I said. "And you've been at him with that marvelous shampoo of yours, haven't you?"

She giggled and walked away and from that day I saw the two of them frequently but at a distance and something like two months went by before I had a chance to talk to her again. She was passing by the surgery as I was coming down the steps and again she grabbed my wrist.

"Mr. Herriot," she said, just as she had done before, "haven't I made a difference to this dog!"

I looked down at Roy with something akin to awe. He had grown and filled out and his coat, no longer yellow but a rich gold, lay in luxuriant shining swathes over the well-fleshed ribs and back. A new, brightly studded collar glittered on his neck and his tail, beautifully fringed, fanned the air gently. He was now a golden retriever in full magnificence. As I stared at him he reared up, plunked his forepaws on my chest, and looked into my face, and in his eyes I read plainly the same calm affection and trust I had seen back in that black, noisome shed.

"Mrs. Donovan," I said softly, "he's the most beautiful dog in Yorkshire." Then, because I knew she was waiting for it, "It's those wonderful condition powders. Whatever do you put in them?"

"Ah, wouldn't you like to know!" She bridled and smiled up at me coquettishly and indeed she was nearer, being kissed at that moment than for many years.

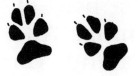

I suppose you could say that

215

was the start of Roy's second life. And as the years passed I often pondered on the beneficent providence which had decreed that an animal which had spent his first twelve months abandoned and unwanted, staring uncomprehendingly into that unchanging, stinking darkness, should be whisked in a moment into an existence of light and movement and love. Because I don't think any dog had it quite so good as Roy from then on.

His diet changed dramatically from odd bread crusts to best stewing steak and biscuit, meaty bones and a bowl of warm milk every evening. And he never missed a thing. Garden fetes, school sports, gymkhanas — he'd be there. I was pleased to note that as time went on Mrs. Donovan seemed to be clocking up an even greater daily mileage. Her expenditure on shoe leather must have been phenomenal, but of course it was absolute pie for Roy — a busy round in the morning, home for a meal then straight out again; it was all go.

Mrs. Donovan didn't confine her activities to the town center; there was a big stretch of common land down by the river where there were seats, and people used to take their dogs for a gallop and she liked to get down there fairly regularly to check on the latest developments on the domestic scene. I often saw Roy loping majestically over the grass among a pack of assorted canines, and when he wasn't doing that he was submitting to being stroked or patted or generally fussed over. He was handsome and he just liked people; it made him irresistible.

It was common knowledge that his mistress had bought a whole selection of brushes and combs of various sizes with which she labored over his coat. Some people said she had a little brush for his teeth, too, and it might have been true, but he certainly wouldn't need his nails clipped — his life on the roads would keep them down.

Mrs. Donovan, too, had her reward; she had a faithful companion by her side every hour of the day and night. But there was more to it than that; she had always had the compulsion to help and heal animals and the salvation of Roy was the high point of her life — a blazing triumph which never dimmed.

I know the memory of it was always fresh because many years later I was sitting on the sidelines at a cricket match and I saw the two of them; the old lady glancing keenly around her, Roy gazing placidly out at the field of play, apparently enjoying every ball. At the end of the match I watched them move away with the dispersing crowd; Roy would be about twelve then and heaven only knows how old Mrs. Donovan must have been, but the big golden animal was trotting along effortlessly and his mistress, a little more bent, perhaps, and her head rather nearer the ground, was going very well.

When she saw me she came over and I felt the familiar tight grip on my wrist.

"Mr. Herriot," she said, and in her eyes the pride was still as warm, the triumph still as bursting new as if it had all happened yesterday.

"Mr. Herriot, haven't I made a difference to this dog!"

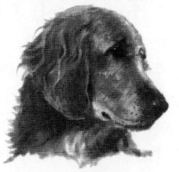

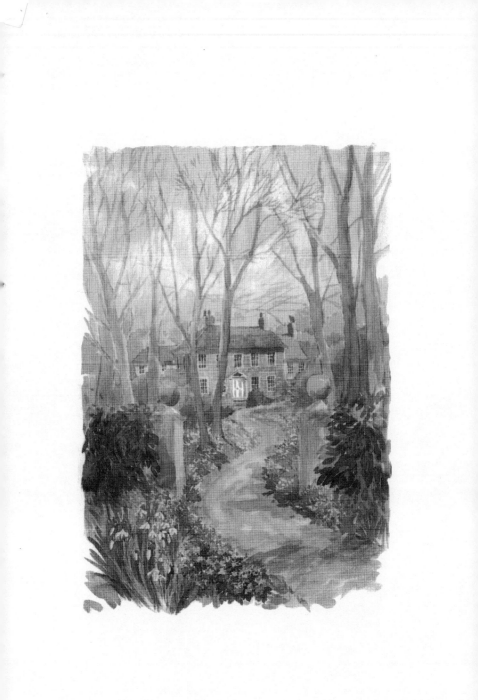

TRICKI WOO

A Judge of Form

I had spent a cold morning out in the fields, and I had just one appointment left. As the road climbed, I began to see the church tower and roofs of Darrowby and, at last, on the edge of the town, the gates of Mrs. Pumphrey's beautiful home lay beckoning. I looked at my watch — twelve noon. Long practice had enabled me to time my visits here just before lunch when I could escape the rigors of country practice and wallow for a little while in the hospitality of the elderly widow who had brightened my life for so long.

As my tires crunched on the gravel of the drive I smiled as Tricki Woo appeared at the window to greet me. He was old now, but he could still get up there to his vantage point and his Pekingese face was split as always by a grin of welcome.

Mounting the steps between the twin pillars of the doorway, I could see that he had left the window and I heard his joyous barking in the hall. Ruth, the long-time maid, answered my ring, beaming with pleasure as Tricki flung himself at my knees.

"Eee, he's glad to see you, Mr. 'erriot," she said and, laying a hand on my arm, "we all are!"

She ushered me into the gracious drawing room, where Mrs. Pumphrey was sitting in an armchair by the fire. She raised her white head from her book and cried out in delight. "Ah, Mr. Herriot, how very very nice! Tricki, isn't it wonderful to have Uncle Herriot visiting again!"

She waved me to the armchair opposite. "I have been expecting you for Tricki's checkup, but before you examine him you must sit down and warm yourself. It is so terribly cold. Ruth, my dear, will you bring Mr. Herriot a glass of sherry. You will say yes, won't you, Mr. Herriot?"

I murmured my thanks. I always said yes to the very special sherry, which came in enormous glasses and was deeply heartening at all times but on cold days in particular. I sank into the cushions and stretched my legs toward the flames which leaped in the fireplace, and as I took my first sip and Ruth deposited a plate of tiny biscuits by my side while the little dog climbed onto my knee, I felt completely at home.

"Tricki has been awfully well since your last visit, Mr. Herriot," Mrs. Pumphrey said. "I know he is always going to be a little stiff with his arthritis but he does get around so well, and his little heart cough is no worse. And, best of all," she clasped her hands together and her eyes widened, "he hasn't gone flop-bott at all. Not once! So perhaps you won't have to squeeze the poor darling."

"Oh no, I won't. Certainly not. I only do that if he really needs it." I had been squeezing Tricki Woo's bottom for many years because of his anal gland trouble so graphically named by his mistress and the little animal had never resented it. I stroked his head as Mrs. Pumphrey went on.

"There is something very interesting I must tell you. As you know, Tricki has always been deeply knowledgeable about horse racing, a wonderful judge of form, and wins nearly all his bets. Well now," she raised a finger and spoke in a confidential murmur, "just recently he has become very interested in greyhound racing!"

"Is that so?"

"Yes, indeed, he has begun to cover the meetings at the Middlesbrough greyhound track and has instructed me to place bets for him and, you know, he has won quite a lot of money already!"

"Gosh!"

"Yes, only this morning Crowther, my chauffeur, collected twelve pounds from the bookmaker after last evening's races."

"Well, well, how wonderful." My heart bled for Joe Downs, the local turf accountant, who must be suffering after losing money on horse racing to a dog for years and then having to pay out on

the greyhounds, too. "Quite re-
markable."

"Isn't it, isn't it!" Mrs. Pumphrey
gave me a radiant smile, then she
became serious. "But I do wonder, Mr. Herriot, just what is responsible for this new interest.
What is your opinion?"

I shook my head gravely. "Difficult to say. Very difficult."

"However, I have a theory," she
said. "Do you think perhaps that
as he grows older he is more
drawn to animals of his own spe-
cies and prefers to bet on doggy
runners like greyhounds?"

"Could be . . . could be . . ."

"And, after all, you would think
with this affinity it would give him
more insight and a better chance
of winning."

"Well, yes, that's possible. That's another point."

Tricki, well aware that we were talking about him, waved his fine tail and looked up at me with his wide grin and lolling tongue.

I settled deeper in the cushions as the sherry began to send warm tendrils through my system. This was a happily familiar situation, listening to Mrs. Pumphrey's recitals of Tricki Woo's activities. She was a kind, highly intelligent, and cultivated lady, admired by all and a benefactress to innumerable charities. She sat on committees and her opinion was sought on many important matters, but where her dog was concerned her conversation never touched on weighty topics, but

was filled with strange and won-
drous things.

She leaned forward in her chair.
"There is something else I would
like to talk to you about, Mr.
Herriot. You know that a Chinese
restaurant has set up in Darrowby?"

"Yes, very nice, too."

She laughed. "But who would
have thought of it? A Chinese
restaurant in a little place like
Darrowby — it's amazing!"

"Very unexpected, I agree. But
this last year or two they have
been popping up all over Britain."

"Yes, but what I want to discuss
with you is that this has affected
Tricki."

"What!"

"Yes, he has been most upset

over the whole business."

"How on earth . . . ?"

"Well, Mr. Herriot," she frowned and gazed at me, solemn-faced, "I told you many years ago and you have always known that Tricki is descended from a long line of Chinese emperors."

"Yes, yes, of course."

"Well, I think I can explain the whole problem if I start at the beginning."

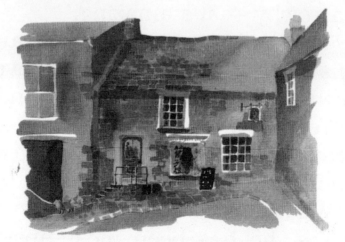

I took a long swallow at my sherry with the pleasant sensation that I was floating away in a dream world. "Please do."

"When the restaurant first opened," she went on, "there was a surprising amount of resentment among some of the local people. They criticized the food and the very nice little Chinese man and his wife, and put it about that there was no place for such a restaurant in Darrowby and that it should not be patronized. Now it so happened that when Tricki and I were out on our little walks, he overheard these remarks in the street, and he was furious."

"Really?"

"Yes, quite affronted. I can tell

233

when he feels like this. He stalks about with an insulted expression and it is so difficult to placate him."

"Dear me, I'm sorry."

"And, after all, one can fully understand how he felt when he heard his own people being denigrated."

"Quite, quite, absolutely — only natural."

"However . . . however, Mr. Herriot," she raised a finger again and gave me a knowing smile, "the clever darling suggested the cure himself."

"He did?"

"Yes, he told me that we ourselves should start to frequent the restaurant and sample their food."

"Ah."

"And that is what we did. I had Crowther drive us there for lunch and we did enjoy it so much. Also, we found we could take the food home all nice and hot in little boxes — what fun! Now that we have started, Crowther often pops out in the evening and brings us our supper and, you know, the restaurant seems quite busy now. I feel we have really helped."

"I'm sure you have," I said, and I meant it. The Lotus Garden, tucked in a corner of the market-place, wasn't much more than a shop front with four small tables inside, and the sight of the gleaming black length of the limousine and uniformed chauffeur parked frequently at its door must have given it a tremendous lift. I was struggling unsuccessfully to picture the locals peering through the window at Mrs. Pumphrey and Tricki eating at one of those tiny tables when she went on.

"I'm so glad you think so. And we have enjoyed it so much. Tricki adores the char sui and my favorite is the chow mein. The little Chinese man is teaching us how to use the chopsticks, too."

I put down my empty glass and dusted the tasty biscuit crumbs from my jacket. I hated to interrupt these sessions and return to reality, but I looked at my watch. "I'm so glad things turned out so nicely, Mrs. Pumphrey, but I think I'd better give the little chap his checkup."

I lifted Tricki onto a chair and palpated his abdomen thoroughly. Nothing wrong there. Then I fished out my stethoscope and listened to his heart and lungs. There was the heart murmur I knew about and some faint bronchitic sounds which I expected. In fact I was totally familiar with all my old friend's internal workings after treating him over the years. Teeth now — maybe could do with another scale next time. Eyes with the beginnings of the lens opacity of the old dog, but not too bad at all.

I turned to Mrs. Pumphrey. Tricki had tablets for his arthritis and the bronchitis but I never elaborated on his ailments to her — too many medical terms upset her. "He's really wonderful for his age, Mrs. Pumphrey. You have his tablets to use when necessary and you know where I am if ever you need me. Just one thing. You have been very good with his diet lately so don't give him too many tidbits — not even extra char sui!"

She giggled and gave me a roguish look. "Oh, please don't scold me, Mr. Herriot. I promise I'll be good." She paused for a moment. "I must mention one more thing with regard to Tricki's arthritis. You know that Hodgkin has been throwing rings for him for years?"

"Yes, I do." Her words raised an image of the dour old gardener under duress casting the rubber rings on the lawn while the little dog, barking in delight, brought them back to him again. Hodgkin, who clearly didn't like dogs, invariably looked utterly fed up and his lips always seemed to be moving as he uttered either to himself or Tricki.

"Well, I thought in view of Tricki's condition that Hodgkin was throwing the rings too far and I told him to throw them for just a few feet. The little darling would have just as much fun with much less exertion."

"I see."

"Unfortunately" — here her expression became disapproving — "Hodgkin has been rather mean about it."

"In what way?"

"I wouldn't have known anything about it," she said, lowering her voice, "but Tricki confided in me."

"Did he really?"

"Yes, he told me that Hodgkin had complained bitterly that it meant he had to bend down a lot more often to pick up the rings and that he had arthritis too. I wouldn't have minded," her voice sank to a whisper, "but Tricki was deeply shocked; he said Hodgkin used the word 'bloody' several times."

"Oh dear, dear, yes, I see the difficulty."

"It has made the whole thing so embarrassing for Tricki. What do you think I should do?"

I nodded sagely and after some cogitation gave my opinion. "I do think, Mrs. Pumphrey, that it would be a good idea to have the throwing sessions less often and for a shorter time. After all, both Tricki and Hodgkin are no longer young."

She gazed at me for a few moments, then smiled fondly. "Oh, thank you, Mr. Herriot, I'm sure you are right, as always. I shall follow your advice."

I looked back as I drove away down the drive. Mrs. Pumphrey and Ruth were smiling and waving from the doorway. Tricki was back at his window, laughing his head off as he barked farewell, the curtains moving with the wagging of his tail. My stomach glowed with sherry and savory biscuits.

Not for the first time I thanked providence for the infinite variety of veterinary practice.

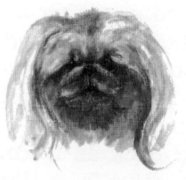

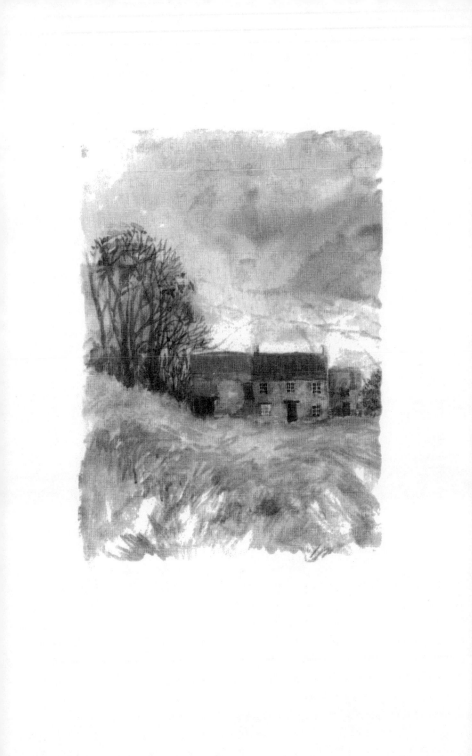

HERMANN

A Happy Ending

"Was there no peace in a vet's life?" I wondered fretfully as I hurried my car along the road to Gilthorpe village. Eight o'clock on a Sunday evening and here I was trailing off to visit a dog ten miles away which, according to Helen who had taken the message, had been ailing for more than a week.

After a long and busy day, I had hoped for a quiet evening, yet here I was back on the treadmill, staring through the windscreen at the roads and the walls which I saw day in, day out. When I left

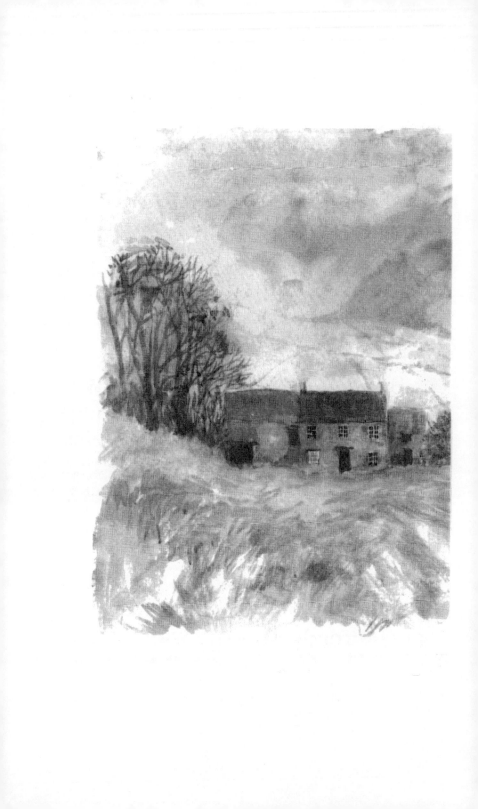

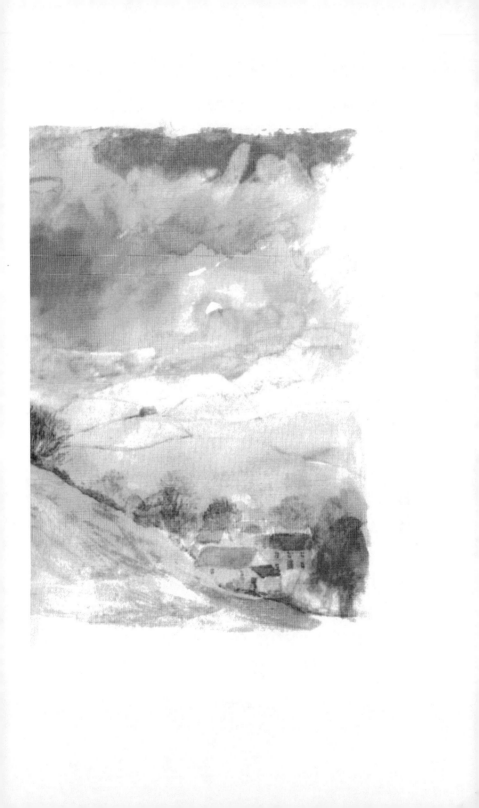

Darrowby the streets of the little town were empty in the gathering dusk and the houses had that tight-shut, comfortable look which raised images of armchairs and pipes and firesides, and now as I saw the lights of the farms winking on the fellsides I could picture the stocksmen dozing contentedly with their feet up.

I had not passed a single car on the darkening road. There was nobody out but Herriot.

I was really sloshing around in my trough of self-pity when I drew up outside a row of gray-stone cottages at the far end of Gilthorpe. Mrs. Cundall, Number 4, Chestnut Row, Helen had written on the slip of paper, and as I opened the gate and stepped through the tiny strip of garden my mind was busy with half-formed ideas of what I was going to say.

My first years' experience in practice had taught me that it did no good at all to remonstrate with people for calling me out at unreasonable times. I knew perfectly well that my words never seemed to get through to them and that they would continue to do so exactly as they had done before, but for all that I had to say something if only to make me feel better.

No need to be rude or ill-mannered, just a firm statement of the position: that vets liked to relax on Sunday evenings just like other people; that we did not mind at all coming out for emergencies but that we did object to having to visit animals which had been ill for a week.

I had my speech fairly well prepared when a little middle-aged woman opened the door.

"Good evening, Mrs. Cundall," I said, slightly tight-lipped.

"Oh, it's Mr. Herriot." She smiled shyly. "We've never met but I've seen you walkin' round Darrowby on market days. Come inside."

The door opened straight into the little low-beamed living room and my first glance took in the shabby furniture and some pictures framed in tarnished gilt when I noticed that the end of the room was partly curtained off.

Mrs. Cundall pulled the curtain aside. In a narrow bed a man was lying, a skeleton-thin man whose eyes looked up at me from hollows in a yellowed face.

"This is my husband, Ron," she said cheerfully, and the man smiled and raised a bony arm from the quilt in greeting.

"And here is your patient — Hermann," she went on, pointing to a little dachshund who sat by the side of the bed.

"Hermann?"

"Yes, we thought it was a good name for a German sausage dog." They both laughed.

"An excellent name. He looks just like a Hermann."

The little animal gazed up at me, bright-eyed and welcoming. I bent down and stroked his head and the pink tongue flickered over my fingers.

I ran my hand over the glossy skin. "He looks very healthy. What's the trouble?"

"Oh, he's fine in himself," Mrs. Cundall replied. "Eats well and everything, but over the last week he's been goin' funny on 'is legs. We weren't all that worried but tonight he sort of flopped down and couldn't get up again."

"I see. I noticed he didn't seem keen to rise when I patted his head." I put my hand under the little dog's body and gently lifted him onto his feet. "Come on, lad," I said. "Come on, Hermann, let's see you walk."

As I encouraged him he took a

few hesitant steps but his hind end swayed progressively and he soon dropped into the sitting position again.

"It's his back, isn't it?" Mrs. Cundall said. "He's strong enough on 'is forelegs."

"That's ma trouble, too," Ron murmured in a soft husky voice, but he was smiling and his wife laughed and patted the arm on the quilt.

I lifted the dog onto my knee. "Yes, the weakness is certainly in the back." I began to palpate the lumbar vertebrae, feeling my way along, watching for any sign of pain.

"Has he hurt 'imself?" Mrs. Cundall asked. "Has somebody hit 'im? We don't usually let

253

him out alone but sometimes he sneaks through the garden gate."

"There's always the possibility of an injury," I said. "But there are other causes." There were indeed — a host of unpleasant possibilities. I did not like the look of this little dog at all. This syndrome was one of the things I hated to encounter in canine practice.

"Can you tell me what you really think?" she said. "I'd like to know."

"Well, an injury could cause hemorrhage or concussion or edema — that's fluid — all affecting his spinal cord. He could even have a fractured vertebra but I don't think so."

"And how about the other causes."

"There's quite a lot. Tumors, bony growths, abscesses, or disks can press on the cord."

"Disks?"

"Yes, little pads of cartilage and fibrous tissue between the vertebrae. In long-bodied dogs like Hermann they sometimes protrude into the spinal canal. In fact I think that is what is causing his symptoms."

Ron's husky voice came again from the bed. "And what's 'is prospects, Mr. Herriot?"

Oh, that was the question. Complete recovery or incurable paralysis. It could be anything. "Very difficult to say at this moment." I replied. "I'll give him an injection and some tablets and we'll see how he goes over the next few days."

I injected an analgesic and some antibiotic and counted out some salicylate tablets into a box. We had no steroids at that time. It was the best I could do.

"Now then, Mr. Herriot." Mrs. Cundall smiled at me eagerly. "Ron has a bottle o' beer every night about this time. Would you like to join 'im?"

"Well . . . it's very kind of you but I don't want to intrude . . ."

"Oh, you're not doing that. We're glad to see you."

She poured two glasses of brown ale, propped her husband up with pillows, and sat down by the bed.

"We're from South Yorkshire, Mr. Herriot," she said.

I nodded. I had noticed the difference from the local accent.

"Aye, we came up here after Ron's accident, eight years ago."

"What was that?"

"I were a miner," Ron said. "Roof fell in on me. I got a broken back, crushed liver, and a lot o' other internal injuries, but two of me mates were killed in the same fall so ah'm lucky to be 'ere." He sipped his beer. "I've survived, but doctor says I'll never walk no more."

"I'm terribly sorry."

"Nay, nay," the husky voice went on. "I count my blessings and I've got a lot to be thankful for. Ah suffer very little and I've got t'best wife in the world."

Mrs. Cundall laughed. "Oh, listen to 'im. But I'm right glad we came to Gilthorpe. We used to spend all our holidays in the Dales. We were great walkers and it was lovely to get away from the smoke and the chimneys. The bedroom in our old house just looked out on a lot o' brick walls but Ron has this big window right by 'im and he can see for miles."

"Yes, of course," I said. "This is a lovely situation." The village was perched on a high ridge on the fellside and that window would command a wide view of the green slopes running down to the river and climbing high to the wildness of the moor on the other side. This sight had beguiled me so often on my rounds and the grassy paths climbing among the airy tops seemed to beckon to me. But they would beckon in vain to Ron Cundall.

"Gettin' Hermann was a good idea, too," he said. "Ah used to feel a bit lonely when t'missus went into Darrowby for shoppin' but the little feller's made all the difference. You're never alone when you've got a dog."

I smiled. "How right you are. What is his age now, by the way?"

"He's six," Ron replied. "Right in the prime o' life, aren't you, old lad." He let his arm fall by the bedside and his hand fondled the sleek ears.

"That seems to be his favorite place."

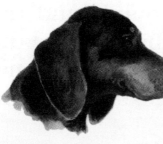

"Aye, it's a funny thing, but 'e allus sits there. T'missus is the one who has to take 'im walks and feeds 'im but he's very faithful to me. He has a basket over there but this is 'is place. I only have to reach down and he's there."

This was something that I had seen on many occasions with disabled people; that their pets stayed close by them as if conscious of their role of comforter and friend.

I finished my beer and got to my feet. Ron looked up at me. "Reckon I'll spin mine out a bit longer." He glanced at his half-full glass. "Ah used to shift about

260

six pints some nights when I went out wi' the lads but you know, I enjoy this one bottle just as much. Strange how things turn out."

His wife bent over him, mock-scolding. "Yes, you've had to right your ways. You're a reformed character, aren't you?"

They both laughed as though it were a stock joke between them.

"Well, thank you for the drink, Mrs. Cundall. I'll look in to see Hermann on Tuesday." I moved toward the door.

As I left I waved to the man in the bed and his wife put her hand on my arm. "We're very grateful to you for comin' out at this time on a Sunday night, Mr. Herriot. We felt awful about callin' you, but you understand it was only today that the little chap started going off his legs like that."

"Oh, of course, of course, please don't worry. I don't mind in the least."

And as I drove through the darkness I knew that I didn't mind — now. My petty irritation had evaporated within two minutes of my entering that house and I was left only with a feeling of humility. If that man back there had a lot to be thankful for, how about me? I had everything. I only wished I could dispel the foreboding I felt about his dog. There was a hint of doom about those symptoms of Hermann and yet I knew I just had to get him right. . . .

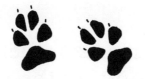

The following Tuesday he looked much the same, possibly a little worse.

"I think I'd better take him back to the surgery for X-ray," I said to Mrs. Cundall. "He doesn't seem to be improving with the treatment."

In the car Hermann curled up happily on the passenger seat.

I had no need to anesthetize him or sedate him when I placed him on our newly acquired X-ray machine. Those hindquarters stayed still all by themselves. A lot too still for my liking.

I was no expert at interpreting X-ray pictures but at least I could be sure there was no fracture of the vertebrae. Also, there was no sign of bony extoses, but I thought I could detect a narrowing of the space between a couple of the vertebrae which would confirm my suspicions of a protrusion of a disk. I could do nothing more than continue with my treatment and hope.

By the end of the week hope had grown very dim. I had supplemented the salicylates with long-standing remedies like tincture of nux vomica and other ancient stimulant drugs, but when I saw Hermann on Saturday he was unable to rise. I tweaked the toes of his hind limbs and was rewarded by a faint reflex movement, but with a sick certainty I knew that complete posterior paralysis was not far away.

A week later I had the unhappy experience of seeing my prognosis confirmed in the most classical way. When I entered the door of the Cundalls' cottage Hermann came to meet me, happy and welcoming in his front end but dragging his hind limbs helplessly behind him.

"Hello, Mr. Herriot." Mrs. Cundall gave me a wan smile and looked down at the little creature stretched froglike on the carpet. "What d'you think of him now?"

I bent and tried the reflexes. Nothing. I shrugged my shoulders, unable to think of anything to say. I looked at the gaunt figure in the bed, the arm outstretched as always on the quilt. "Good morning, Ron," I said as cheerfully as I could, but there was no reply. The face was averted, looking out of the window. I walked over to the bed. Ron's eyes were staring fixedly at the glorious panorama of the moor and fell, at the pebbles of the river, white in the early sunshine, at the crisscross of the gray walls against the green. His face was expressionless. It was as though he did not know I was there.

I went back to his wife. I don't think I have ever felt more miserable.

"Is he annoyed with me?" I whispered.

"No, no, no, it's this." She held

266

out a newspaper. "It's upset him something awful."

I looked at the printed page. There was a large picture at the top, a picture of a dachshund exactly like Hermann. This dog, too, was paralyzed but its hind end was supported by a little four-wheeled bogie. In the picture it appeared to be sporting with its mistress. In fact it looked normal except for those wheels.

Ron seemed to hear the rustle of the paper because his head came round quickly. "What d'ye think of that, Mr. Herriot? D'ye agree with it?"

"Well . . . I don't really know, Ron. I don't like the look of it, but I suppose the lady in the picture thought it was the only thing to do."

"Aye, maybe." The husky voice trembled. "But ah don't want Hermann to finish up like that." The arm dropped by the side of the bed and his fingers felt around on the carpet, but the little dog was still splayed out near the door. "It's 'opeless now, Mr. Herriot, isn't it?"

"Well, it was a black lookout from the beginning," I said. "These cases are so difficult. I'm very sorry."

"Nay, I'm not blamin' you," he said. "You've done what ye could, same as vet for that dog in the picture did what 'e could. But it was no good, was it? What do we do now — put 'im down?"

"No, Ron, forget about that just now. Sometimes paralysis cases

268

just recover on their own after many weeks. We must carry on. At this moment I honestly cannot say there is no hope."

I paused for a moment, then turned to Mrs. Cundall. "One of the problems is the dog's natural functions. You'll have to carry him out into the garden for that. I'm sure you'll soon learn how to cope."

"Oh, of course, of course," she replied. "I'll do anything. As long as there's some hope."

"There is, I assure you, there is."

But on the way back to the surgery the thought hammered in my brain. That hope was very slight. Spontaneous recovery did sometimes occur but Hermann's condition was extreme. I repressed a groan as I thought of the nightmarish atmosphere which had begun to surround my dealings with the Cundalls. The paralyzed man and the paralyzed dog. And why did that picture have to appear in the paper just at this very time? Every veterinary surgeon knows the feeling that fate has loaded the scales against him, and it weighed on me despite the bright sunshine spreading into the car.

However, I kept going back every few days. Sometimes I took a couple of bottles of brown ale along in the evening and drank them with Ron. He and his wife were always cheerful but the little dog never showed the slightest

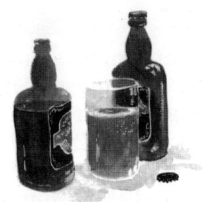

sign of improvement. He still had to pull his useless hind limbs after him when he came to greet me, and although he always returned to his station by his master's bed, nuzzling up into Ron's hand, I was beginning to resign myself to the certainty that one day that arm would come down from the quilt and Hermann would not be there.

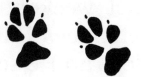

It was on one of these visits that

I noticed an unpleasant smell as I entered the house. There was something familiar about it.

I sniffed and the Cundalls looked at each other guiltily. There was a silence and then Ron spoke.

"It's some medicine ah've been givin' Hermann. Stinks like 'ell but it's supposed to be good for dogs."

"Oh yes?"

"Aye, well . . ." His fingers twitched uncomfortably on the bedclothes. "It was Bill Noakes put me on to it. He's an old mate o' mine — we used to work down t'pit together — and he came to visit me last weekend. Keeps a few whippets, does Bill. Knows a lot about dogs and 'e sent me this stuff along for Hermann."

272

Mrs. Cundall went to the cupboard and sheepishly presented me with a plain bottle. I removed the cork and as the horrid stench rose up to me my memory became suddenly clear. Asafetida, a common constituent of quack medicines before the war and still lingering on the shelves of occasional chemist shops and in the medicine chests of people who liked to doctor their own animals.

I had never prescribed the stuff myself but it was supposed to be beneficial in horses with colic and dogs with digestive troubles. My own feeling had always been that its popularity had been due solely to the assumption that anything which stank as badly as that

must have some magical proper-
ties, but one thing I knew for sure
was that it could not possibly do
anything for Hermann.

I replaced the cork. "So you're
giving him this, eh?"

Ron nodded. "Aye, three times
a day. He doesn't like it much,
but Bill Noakes has great faith in
it. Cured hundreds o' dogs with
it, 'e says." The deep-sunk eyes
looked at me with a silent appeal.

"Well, fine, Ron," I said. "You
carry on. Let's hope it does the
trick."

I knew the asafetida couldn't do
any harm and since my treatment had proved useless I was in
no position to turn haughty. But
my main concern was that these
two nice people had been given a

glimmer of hope, and I wasn't going to blot it out.

Mrs. Cundall smiled and Ron's expression relaxed. "That's grand, Mr. Herriot," he said. "Ah'm glad ye don't mind. I can dose the little feller myself. It's summat for me to do."

It was about a week after the commencement of the new treatment that I called in at the Cundalls' as I was passing through Gilthorpe.

"How are you today, Ron?" I asked.

"Champion, Mr. Herriot, champion." He always said that, but today there was a new eagerness in his face. He reached down and lifted his dog onto the bed. "Look 'ere."

I pinched the little paw between his fingers and there was a faint but definite retraction of the leg. I almost fell over in my haste to grab at the other foot. The result was the same.

"My God, Ron," I gasped, "the reflexes are coming back."

He laughed his soft, husky laugh. "Bill Noakes's stuff's working, isn't it?"

A gush of emotions, mainly professional shame and wounded pride, welled in me, but it was only for a moment. "Yes, Ron," I replied, "it's working. No doubt about it."

He stared up at me. "Then Hermann's going to be all right."

"Well, it's early days yet, but that's the way it looks to me."

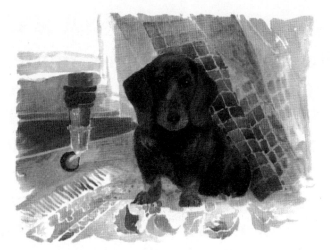

It was several weeks more before the little dachshund was back to normal and of course it was a fairly typical case of spontaneous recovery with nothing whatever to do with the asafetida or indeed with my own efforts. Even now, thirty years later, when I treat these puzzling back conditions with steroids, I wonder how many of them would have recovered without my aid. Quite a number, I imagine.

Sadly, despite the modern drugs, we still have our failures, and I always regard a successful termination with profound relief.

But that feeling of relief has never been stronger than it was with Hermann, and I can recall vividly my final call at the cottage in Gilthorpe. As it happened it was around the same time as my first visit — eight o'clock in the evening, and when Mrs. Cundall ushered me in, the little dog bounded joyously up to me before returning to his post by the bed.

"Well, that's a lovely sight," I said. "He can gallop like a racehorse now."

Ron dropped his hand down and stroked the sleek head. "Aye,

isn't it grand. By heck, it's been a worryin' time."

"Well, I'll be going." I gave Hermann a farewell pat. "I just looked in on my way home to make sure all was well. I don't need to come anymore now."

"Nay, nay," Ron said. "Don't rush off. You've time to have a bottle o' beer with me before ye go."

I sat down by the bed and Mrs. Cundall gave us our glasses before pulling up a chair for herself. It was exactly like that first night. I poured my beer and looked at the two of them. Their faces glowed with friendliness and I marveled because my part in Hermann's salvation had been anything but heroic.

In their eyes everything I had done must have seemed bumbling and ineffectual and in fact they must have been convinced that all would have been lost if Ron's old chum from the coalface had not stepped in and effortlessly put things right.

At best they could only regard me as an amiable fathead and all the explanations and protestations in the world would not alter that. But though my ego had been bruised I did not really care. I was witnessing a happy ending instead of a tragedy, and that was more important than petty self-justification. I made a mental resolve never to say anything which might spoil their picture of this triumph.

I was about to take my first sip when Mrs. Cundall spoke up. "This is your last visit, Mr. Herriot, and all's ended well. I think we ought to drink some sort o' toast."

"I agree," I said. "Let's see, what shall it be? Ah yes, I've got it." I raised my glass. "Here's to Bill Noakes."

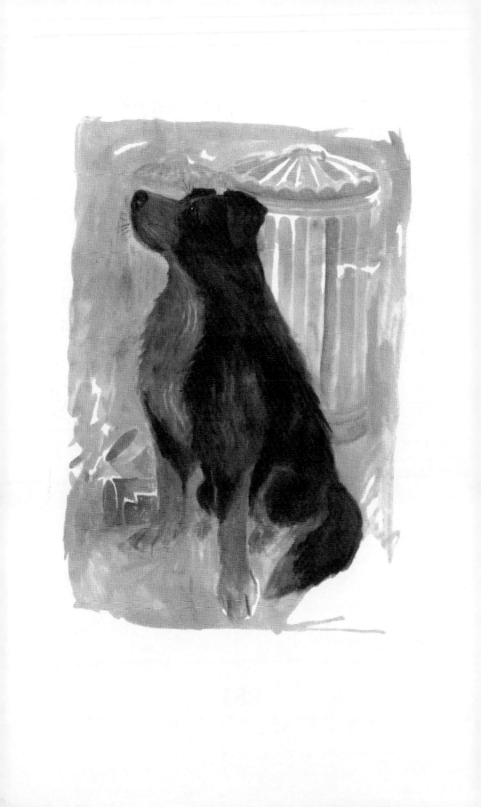

BRANDY

The Dustbin Dog

In the semidarkness of the surgery passage I thought it was a hideous growth dangling from the side of the dog's face, but as he came closer I saw that it was only a condensed milk can. Not that condensed milk cans are commonly found sprouting from dogs' cheeks, but I was relieved because I knew I was dealing with Brandy again.

I hoisted him onto the table. "Brandy, you've been at the dustbin again."

The big brown and black mutt

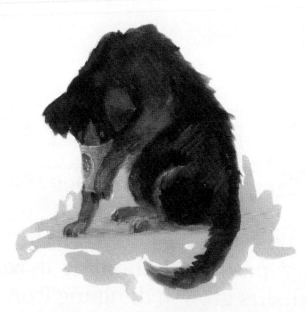

gave me an apologetic grin and did his best to lick my face. He couldn't manage it since his tongue was jammed inside the can, but he made up for it by a furious wagging of tail and rear end.

"Oh, Mr. Herriot, I am sorry to trouble you again." Mrs. Westby, his attractive young mistress, smiled ruefully. "He just won't keep out of that dustbin. Sometimes the children and I can get the cans off ourselves but this one is stuck fast. His tongue is trapped under the lid."

"Yes . . . yes . . ." I eased my finger along the jagged edge of the metal. "It's a bit tricky, isn't it? We don't want to cut his mouth."

As I reached for a pair of forceps I thought of the many other occasions when I had done something like this for Brandy. He was one of my patients, a huge, lolloping, slightly goofy animal, but his dustbin raiding was becoming an obsession.

He liked to fish out a can and lick out the tasty remnants, but his licking was carried out with such dedication that he burrowed deeper and deeper until he got stuck. Again and again he had been freed by his family or myself from fruit salad cans, corned beef cans, baked bean cans, soup cans. There didn't seem to be any kind of can he didn't like.

I gripped the edge of the lid with my forceps and gently bent it back along its length until I was able to lift it away from the tongue. An instant later, that tongue was slobbering all over my cheek as Brandy expressed his delight and thanks.

"Get away, you daft dog!" I said, laughing, as I held the panting face away from me.

"Yes, come down, Brandy," Mrs. Westby hauled him from the table and spoke sharply. "It's all very fine making a fuss now, but you're becoming a nuisance with this business. It will have to stop."

The scolding had no effect on the lashing tail and I saw that his mistress was smiling. You just couldn't help liking Brandy, because he was a great ball of affection and tolerance without an ounce of malice in him.

I had seen the Westby children — there were three girls and a boy — carrying him around by the legs, upside down, or pushing him in a pram, sometimes dressed in baby clothes. Those youngsters played all sorts of games with him, but he suffered them all with good humor. In fact I am sure he enjoyed them.

Brandy had other idiosyncrasies apart from his fondness for dustbins.

I was attending the Westby cat at their home one afternoon when I noticed the dog acting strangely. Mrs. Westby was sitting knitting in an armchair while the oldest girl squatted on the hearth rug with me and held the cat's head.

It was when I was searching my pockets for my thermometer that I noticed Brandy slinking into the room. He wore a furtive air as he moved across the carpet and sat down with studied carelessness in front of his mistress. After a few moments he began to work his rear end gradually up the front of the chair toward her knees. Absently she took a hand away from her knitting and

288

pushed him down but he immediately restarted his backward
ascent. It was an extraordinary
mode of progression, his hips
moving in very slow rumba
rhythm as he elevated them inch
by inch, and all the time the
handsome face was blank and
innocent as though nothing at all
was happening.

Fascinated, I stopped hunting
for my thermometer and watched.
Mrs. Westby was absorbed in an
intricate part of her knitting and
didn't seem to notice that
Brandy's bottom was now firmly
parked on her shapely knees,
which were clad in blue jeans.
The dog paused as though ac-
knowledging that phase one had
been successfully completed,

then ever so gently he began to consolidate his position, pushing his way up the front of the chair with his forelimbs until at one time he was almost standing on his head.

It was at that moment, just when one final backward heave would have seen the great dog ensconced on her lap, that Mrs. Westby finished the tricky bit of knitting and looked up.

"Oh, really, Brandy, you are silly!" She put a hand on his rump and sent him slithering disconsolately to the carpet where he lay and looked at her with liquid eyes.

"What was all that about?" I asked.

Mrs. Westby laughed. "Oh, it's

these old blue jeans. When Brandy first came here as a tiny puppy I spent hours nursing him on my knee and I used to wear the jeans a lot then. Ever since, even though he's a grown dog, the very sight of the things makes him try to get on my knee."

"But he doesn't jump up?"

"Oh, no," she said. "He's tried it and got pushed off. He knows perfectly well I can't have a huge dog in my lap."

"So now it's the stealthy approach, eh?"

She giggled. "That's right. When I'm preoccupied — knitting or reading — sometimes he manages to get nearly all the way up, and if he's been playing in the mud he makes an awful mess and I have to go and change. That's when he really does receive a scolding."

A patient like Brandy added color to my daily round. When I was walking my own dog I often saw him playing in the fields by the river. One particularly hot day, many of the dogs were taking to the water either to chase sticks or just to cool off, but whereas they glided in and swam off sedately, Brandy's approach was unique.

I watched as he ran up to the riverbank, expecting him to pause before entering. But instead he launched himself outward, legs splayed in a sort of swallow dive, and hung for a moment in the air rather like a flying fox before splashing thunderously into the depths. To me it was the action of a completely happy extrovert.

On the following day in those same fields I witnessed something even more extraordinary. There is a little children's playground in one corner — a few swings, a roundabout, and a slide. Brandy was disporting himself on the slide.

For this activity he had assumed an uncharacteristic gravity of expression and stood calmly in the line of children. When his turn came he mounted the steps, slid down the metal slope, all dignity and importance, then took a staid walk round to rejoin the line.

The little boys and girls who

were his companions seemed to take him for granted, but I found it difficult to tear myself away. I could have watched him all day.

I often smiled to myself when I thought of Brandy's antics, but I didn't smile when Mrs. Westby brought him into the surgery a few months later. His bounding ebullience had disappeared and he dragged himself along the passage to the consulting room.

As I lifted him onto the table I noticed that he had lost a lot of weight.

"Now, what is the trouble, Mrs. Westby?" I asked.

She looked at me worriedly. "He's been off color for a few days now, listless and coughing and not eating very well, but this

294

morning he seems quite ill and you can see he's starting to pant."

"Yes . . . yes . . ." As I inserted the thermometer I watched the rapid rise and fall of the rib cage and noted the gaping mouth and anxious eyes. "He does look very sorry for himself."

His temperature was 104°F. I took out my stethoscope and listened to his chest. I have heard of an old Scottish doctor describing a seriously ill patient's chest as sounding like a "kist o' whustles" and that just about described Brandy's. Wheezes, squeaks, and bubblings — they were all there against a background of labored respiration.

I put the stethoscope back in

my pocket. "He's got pneumonia."

"Oh dear." Mrs. Westby reached out and touched the heaving chest. "That's bad, isn't it?"

"Yes, I'm afraid so."

"But . . ." She gave me an appealing glance. "I understand it isn't so fatal since the new drugs came out."

I hesitated. "Yes, that's quite right. In humans and most animals the sulfa drugs and now penicillin have changed the picture completely, but I'm afraid dogs are still very difficult to cure."

Thirty years later it is still the same. Even with all the armory of antibiotics which followed penicillin — streptomycin, the tetracyclines, and synthetics, and the new nonantibiotic drugs and steroids — I still hate to see pneumonia in a dog.

"But you don't think it's hopeless?" Mrs. Westby asked, her face full of anxiety.

"No, no, not at all. I'm just warning you that so many dogs don't respond to treatment when they should. But Brandy is young and strong. He must stand a fair chance. I wonder what started this off, anyway."

"Oh, I think I know, Mr. Herriot. He had a swim in the river about a week ago. I try to keep him out of the water in this cold weather but if he sees a stick floating he just takes a dive into the middle. You've seen him — it's one of the funny little things he does."

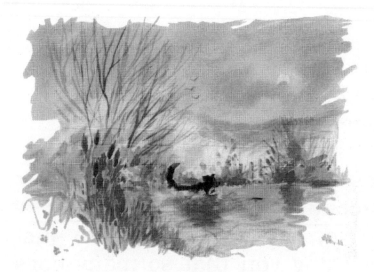

"Yes, I know. And was he shivery afterward?"

"He was. I walked him straight home, but it was such a freezing cold day. I could feel him trembling so I dried him down."

I nodded. "That would be the cause, all right. Anyway, let's start his treatment. I'm going to give him this injection of penicillin and I'll call at your house tomorrow to repeat it. He's not

well enough to come to the surgery."

"Very well, Mr. Herriot. And is
there anything else?"

"Yes, there is. I want you to
make him what we call a pneumonia jacket. Cut two holes in an
old blanket for his forelegs and
stitch him into it along his back.
You can use an old sweater if you
like, but he must have his chest
warmly covered. Only let him out
in the garden for necessities."

I called and repeated the injection on the following day. There
wasn't much change. I injected
him for four more days and the
realization came to me sadly that
Brandy was like so many of the
others — he wasn't responding.
The temperature did drop a little

but he ate hardly anything and grew gradually thinner.

As the days passed and he continued to cough and pant and to sink deeper into a blank-eyed lethargy, I was forced more and more to a conclusion which, a few weeks ago, would have seemed impossible; that this happy, bounding animal was going to die.

But Brandy didn't die. He survived. You couldn't put it any better than that. His temperature came down and his appetite improved and he climbed onto a plateau of twilight existence where he seemed content to stay.

"He isn't Brandy anymore," Mrs. Westby said one morning a few weeks later when I called in.

Her eyes filled with tears.

I shook my head. "No, I'm afraid he isn't. Are you giving him the halibut-liver oil?"

"Yes, every day. But nothing seems to do him any good. Why is he like this, Mr. Herriot?"

"Well, he has recovered from a really virulent pneumonia, but it's left him with a chronic pleurisy, adhesions, and probably other kinds of lung damage. It looks as though he's just stuck there."

She dabbed at her eyes. "It breaks my heart to see him like this. He's only five, but he's like an old, old dog. He was so full of life, too." She sniffed and blew her nose. "When I think of how I used to scold him for getting into the dustbins and muddying up my

301

jeans. How I wish he would do some of his funny old tricks now."

I thrust my hands deep into my pockets. "Never does anything like that now, eh?"

"No, no, just hangs about the house. Doesn't even want to go for a walk."

As I watched, Brandy rose from his place in the corner and pottered slowly over to the fire. He stood there for a moment, gaunt and dead-eyed, and he seemed to notice me for the first time because the end of his tail gave a brief twitch before he coughed, groaned, and flopped down on the hearth rug.

Mrs. Westby was right. He was like a very old dog.

"Do you think he'll always be

like this?" she asked.

I shrugged. "We can only hope."

But as I got into my car and drove away I really didn't have much hope. I had seen calves with lung damage after bad pneumonias. They recovered but were called "bad doers" because they remained thin and listless for the rest of their lives. Doctors, too, had plenty of "chesty" people on their books; they were, more or less, in the same predicament.

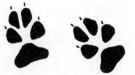

Weeks and then months went by and the only time I saw Brandy was when Mrs. Westby was walking him on his lead. I always had the impression that he was reluctant to move and his mistress had to stroll along very slowly so that he could keep up with her. The sight of him saddened me when I thought of the lolloping dog of old, but I told myself that at least I had saved his life. I could do no more for him now and I made a determined effort to push him out of my mind.

In fact I tried to forget Brandy and managed to do so fairly well until one afternoon in February. On the previous night I felt I had been through the fire. I had treated a colicky horse until 4:00 A.M. and was crawling into bed, comforted by the knowledge that the animal was settled down and free from pain, when I was called to a calving. I had managed to produce a large live calf from a small heifer, but the effort had drained the last of my strength and when I got home it was too late to return to bed.

Plowing through the morning round I was so tired that I felt disembodied, and at lunch Helen watched me anxiously as my head nodded over my food. There were a few dogs in the waiting room at two o'clock and I dealt with them mechanically, peering through half-closed eyelids. By the time I reached my last patient I was almost asleep on my feet. In fact I had the feeling that I wasn't there at all.

"Next, please." I mumbled as I pushed open the waiting room

door and stood back waiting for the usual sight of a dog being led out to the passage.

But this time there was a big difference. There was a man in the doorway all right and he had a little poodle with him, but the thing that made my eyes snap wide open was that the dog was walking upright on his hind limbs.

I knew I was half-asleep but surely I wasn't seeing things. I stared down at the dog, but the picture hadn't changed — the little creature strutted through the doorway, chest out, head up, as erect as a soldier.

"Follow me, please," I said hoarsely and set off over the tiles to the consulting room. Halfway along I just had to turn round to check the evidence of my eyes and it was just the same — the poodle, still on his hind legs, marching along unconcernedly at his master's side.

The man must have seen the bewilderment on my face because he burst suddenly into a roar of laughter.

"Don't worry, Mr. Herriot," he said. "This little dog was circus trained before I got him as a pet. I like to show off his little tricks. This one really startles people."

"You can say that again," I said breathlessly. "It nearly gave me heart failure."

The poodle wasn't ill, he just wanted his nails clipped. I smiled as I hoisted him onto the table and began to ply the clippers.

"I suppose he won't want his hind claws doing," I said. "He'll have worn them down himself." I was glad to find I had recovered sufficiently to attempt a little joke.

However, by the time I had finished, the old lassitude had taken over again and I felt ready to fall down as I showed man and dog to the front door.

I watched the little animal trotting away down the street — in the orthodox manner this time — and it came to me suddenly that it had been a long time since I had seen a dog doing something unusual and amusing. Like the things Brandy used to do.

A wave of gentle memories flowed through me as I leaned

wearily against the door post and closed my eyes. When I opened them I saw Brandy coming round the corner of the street with Mrs. Westby. His nose was entirely obscured by a large red tomato soup can and he strained madly at the leash and whipped his tail when he saw me.

It was certainly a hallucination this time. I was looking into the past. I really ought to go to bed immediately. But I was still rooted to the door post when the big dog bounded up the steps, made an attempt, aborted by the soup can, to lick my face, and contented himself with cocking a convivial leg against the bottom step.

I stared into Mrs. Westby's radiant face. "What . . . what . . . ?"

With her sparkling eyes and wide smile she looked more attractive than ever. "Look, Mr. Herriot, look! He's better, he's better!"

In an instant I was wide awake. "And I . . . I suppose you'll want me to get that can off him?"

"Oh, yes, yes, please!"

It took all my strength to lift him onto the table. He was heavier now than before his illness. I reached for the familiar forceps and began to turn the jagged edges of the can outward from the nose and mouth. Tomato soup must have been one of his favorites because he was really deeply embedded and it took some time before I was able to slide the can from his face.

I fought off his slobbering at-
tack. "He's back in the dustbins,
I see."

"Yes, he is, quite regularly. I've
pulled several cans off him myself. And he goes sliding with the
children, too." She smiled happily.

Thoughtfully I took my stethoscope from the pocket of my white
coat and listened to his lungs.
They were wonderfully clear. A
slight roughness here and there,
but the old cacophony had gone.

I leaned on the table and looked
at the great dog with a mixture
of thankfulness and incredulity.
He was as before, boisterous and
full of the joy of living. His tongue
lolled in a happy grin and the sun

glinted through the surgery window on his sleek brown and black coat.

"But Mr. Herriot," Mrs. Westby's eyes were wide, "how on earth has this happened? How has he got better?"

"*Vis medicatrix naturae,*" I replied in tones of deep respect.

"I beg your pardon?"

"The healing power of nature. Something no veterinary surgeon can compete with when it decides to act."

"I see. And you can never tell when this is going to happen?"

"No."

For a few seconds we were silent as we stroked the dog's head, ears, and flanks.

"Oh, by the way," I said. "Has

312

he shown any renewed interest in the blue jeans?"

"Oh my word, yes! They're in the washing machine at this very moment. Absolutely covered in mud. Isn't it marvelous!"

We hope you have enjoyed this Large Print book. Other G.K. Hall & Co. or Chivers Press Large Print books are available at your library or directly from the publishers.

For more information about current and upcoming titles, please call or write, without obligation, to:

G.K. Hall & Co.
P.O. Box 159
Thorndike, Maine 04986
USA
Tel. (800) 223-2336

OR

Chivers Press Limited
Windsor Bridge Road
Bath BA2 3AX
England
Tel. (0225) 335336

All our Large Print titles are designed for easy reading, and all our books are made to last.